THE SECRET HEALTH PROTOCOL

The Practical Plan to Eliminate Inflammation, Restore Energy, and Reclaim Your Health

The Hidden Architecture

Healing begins the moment you stop fighting your body and start listening to it

Table of Contents

Part I. The Hidden Causes of Chronic Illness

Before you can fix something, you need to see it clearly. That's the hardest part of modern health: most of what's making you sick doesn't look dangerous on the surface. It's not the car accident or the broken bone. It's the quiet drip of stress hormones day after day. The additives hiding in your food. The low-grade inflammation simmering under your skin. These aren't events you can point to; they're environments you live in. And because you live in them, you stop noticing them — until your body forces you to.

The problem isn't that your body is broken. It's that it's responding, perfectly, to the conditions you've been living under. Constant exposure to processed food, hidden chemicals, chronic stress, and disrupted sleep has taught your body to stay in fight-or-flight mode. Over time, this becomes your "normal," even though it's not what your biology was built for. Fatigue, brain fog, joint aches, stubborn weight, mood swings — these aren't random symptoms. They're signals. And the signals all point in one direction: the body is inflamed and overloaded.

Mainstream medicine rarely talks about this bigger picture. You go to the doctor with fatigue, and they check your labs. If nothing shows up, you're told everything is "fine." If something is off, you get a prescription. Either way, the deeper question — *why is the system inflamed in the first place?* — is rarely answered. The result? People manage symptoms for years without ever addressing the root.

This part of the book is about shining a light on those hidden roots. We're going to break down the silent forces that shape your daily energy, your hormones, and even your mood — forces that most people never realize are at play. You'll learn how common foods trigger inflammation without obvious reactions, how environmental toxins disrupt hormonal balance, and why chronic stress quietly rewires your biology.

The goal here isn't to scare you. It's to give you clarity. Because when you see the true causes, you can finally take action that works. And action doesn't mean extremes — no crash detoxes, no living on celery juice, no chasing miracle supplements. It means understanding what's draining you, removing what you can, and giving your body what it's been missing so it can start doing what it was built to do: heal.

By the end of this part, you'll understand why you feel the way you do — and, more importantly, you'll know exactly where to begin to change it.

The Hidden Epidemic of Fatigue, Brain Fog, and Inflammation

You can feel it in the mornings when you wake up already tired. You feel it when you reach for coffee just to stay functional, and again in the afternoons when your mind seems to slow to a crawl. You feel it when you can't remember simple details or when your body aches even though you did nothing extreme the day before. This quiet, creeping exhaustion is not rare anymore — it's so common that many people think it's normal.

But what's happening under the surface is far from normal. Fatigue, brain fog, and chronic inflammation have become some of the most widespread, underrecognized health problems of our time. Millions of people are walking around every day in a state of low-grade dysfunction, wondering why they can't lose weight, why their mood is unpredictable, or why their body seems to age faster than it should. It isn't laziness. It isn't a lack of willpower. It's biology reacting to an environment that has shifted dramatically in just a few decades.

Why This Epidemic Is "Hidden"

The biggest reason this crisis flies under the radar is that it rarely shows up in standard medical tests. When your bloodwork looks "fine," you are often told nothing is wrong. Yet you still feel exhausted. The truth is, the most important drivers of fatigue and brain fog — subtle hormonal shifts, chronic low-grade inflammation, disruptions in gut health — don't always produce abnormalities on basic lab work. They're functional imbalances rather than overt diseases. And because they develop slowly, you might adapt to them, thinking, *maybe this is just getting older.*

Another reason it stays hidden is cultural. We've normalized being overworked, underslept, overstimulated, and undernourished. It's become common to joke about brain fog or exhaustion, but the normalization hides how serious the issue is. Constant fatigue isn't just an inconvenience; it is a signal that your body is running on emergency power.

The Inflammation Connection

At the center of this epidemic lies inflammation — a biological process that is both necessary and potentially destructive. Inflammation is your body's defense mechanism, meant to fight infection or heal injuries. But when the signal never turns off, it becomes harmful. This chronic, low-level inflammation affects every major system in your body. It disrupts your hormones, weakens your immune system, slows your metabolism, and clouds your thinking.

What makes chronic inflammation tricky is that you can't always see or feel it directly. It doesn't announce itself with sharp pain or obvious swelling. It's more like background noise: subtle, constant, and easily overlooked until it leads to something bigger — persistent fatigue, joint pain, digestive problems, or even conditions like insulin resistance.

Brain Fog: The Silent Partner of Fatigue

Alongside inflammation comes brain fog — that frustrating inability to focus or think clearly. It's more than forgetfulness; it's a sense of mental heaviness that lingers no matter how much coffee you drink. This fog is tied to inflammatory processes in the brain itself, as well as fluctuations in blood sugar, disrupted sleep, and the overstimulation of modern life. When your nervous system is stuck in overdrive, your brain prioritizes survival over higher-level thinking. The result? Difficulty concentrating, remembering details, or staying emotionally regulated.

These symptoms often create a ripple effect through everyday life. Fatigue makes it harder to prepare balanced meals or stick to routines. Brain fog interferes with work performance and personal relationships. Inflammation itself can lead to cravings for comfort foods, poor sleep, and more stress, which in turn feed the cycle further. People end up blaming themselves, thinking they lack discipline, when in reality their bodies are responding exactly as they were designed to under chronic stress and toxic load.

The Role of Modern Lifestyles

Modern living amplifies these problems in ways previous generations never faced. The typical diet is high in refined carbohydrates, industrial seed oils, and additives that disrupt the gut and promote systemic inflammation. At the same time, stress has become constant rather than occasional. Most people are tethered to their devices, exposed to artificial light late into the night, and cut off from natural rhythms that guide hormonal balance. Even small things — like sitting for long periods or living in poorly ventilated spaces — add up to create an internal environment that keeps the immune system on alert.

These aren't isolated factors. When combined, they overwhelm the body's ability to repair and recover. The nervous system shifts into a chronic state of vigilance. Hormones like cortisol and insulin spike, then crash. The gut barrier weakens, letting inflammatory molecules circulate more freely. Over months and years, this pattern becomes self-perpetuating.

Why So Many Solutions Fall Short

The health industry is full of quick fixes aimed at these symptoms, but most fail because they treat isolated problems rather than the interconnected system. A stimulant might boost energy for a few hours but does nothing for inflammation. A fad diet might produce short-term weight loss but worsen hormonal balance or gut health. Even well-intentioned supplements can backfire if they are added to a body still overloaded by toxins and stress. Without addressing the root environment driving these issues, temporary relief is all most people get.

Recognizing the Signals

Learning to recognize the body's subtle warning signs is crucial. Constant tiredness after meals, trouble waking up rested, difficulty concentrating, mood swings, or unexplained joint stiffness are not random annoyances. They are clues. When seen together, they form a clear picture of chronic inflammation and dysregulation. Identifying these patterns early allows you to intervene before they escalate into more serious health challenges.

The Path Forward

Breaking free from this hidden epidemic requires a shift in perspective. Rather than searching for a single miracle food or supplement, the solution comes from creating conditions where the body can restore its own balance. That means removing the inputs that fuel inflammation and giving the body the nutrients, rest, and rhythms it needs to heal. It is less about adding more complexity to your life and more about stripping away what silently harms you.

This book exists to guide that process. By understanding the connections between fatigue, brain fog, and inflammation, you gain the clarity to act with confidence. The goal isn't perfection but steady progress toward an internal environment that supports energy and resilience instead of draining them. The next chapters will help you identify the specific triggers at play in your own life and begin building a protocol tailored to your body's needs, one step at a time.

Why Symptom-Based Medicine Failed You

Most people enter the healthcare system because they want relief. They feel tired, achy, or foggy, and they hope a doctor can identify the cause and fix it. The problem is that modern medicine isn't built to search for root causes — it is built to manage symptoms. If you have high blood pressure, you get medication to lower it. If you have pain, you get something to mask it. If you have trouble sleeping, you might be prescribed a pill to help you drift off. The immediate discomfort may improve, but the underlying imbalance remains untouched.

This system works reasonably well in emergencies. If you break a bone, suffer a heart attack, or develop an acute infection, modern medicine can save your life. Where it fails is in the world of chronic, subtle dysfunction — the kind that builds up over years. Conditions like fatigue, brain fog, and low-grade inflammation don't usually appear as one dramatic event. They creep in slowly, and standard medical approaches rarely address them because they don't fit neatly into diagnostic boxes.

The Focus on Symptoms Instead of Systems

When you visit a doctor, the focus is almost always on what can be measured in that moment: lab results, vital signs, visible symptoms. If nothing alarming shows up, you may be told everything is normal, even though you know your energy and mental clarity are far from normal. If something is slightly off, you might receive a prescription to control that specific marker without investigating why it became imbalanced in the first place.

This isn't entirely the fault of individual doctors. It's the structure of the system itself. Insurance companies reward quick visits and measurable outcomes. Pharmaceutical companies drive research toward drugs that manage markers rather than cure root causes. As a result, the average patient spends years cycling through appointments, tests, and prescriptions without ever getting to the real reason behind their symptoms.

How This Approach Keeps You Stuck

Treating symptoms in isolation can even worsen long-term health. For example, someone with joint pain might be prescribed anti-inflammatory drugs that ease pain temporarily but irritate the gut lining, leading to further inflammation over time. Someone with fatigue might be given stimulants that help for a few hours but disrupt sleep, compounding the original problem. Each band-aid creates new imbalances that add to the body's burden instead of lifting it.

Over time, this creates a frustrating loop: new symptoms lead to new medications, which lead to new side effects, which then lead to more appointments. It's no wonder so many people feel like they are fighting their bodies rather than working with them.

Looking beyond symptoms means looking at the body as an interconnected system rather than a collection of separate parts. Fatigue, brain fog, weight gain, and hormonal imbalances are rarely isolated issues. They are signals of stress somewhere in the network — gut health affecting the brain, chronic stress affecting hormones, or nutrient deficiencies impacting energy production. When one system struggles, others compensate, and that compensation eventually leads to more symptoms.

The shift toward root-cause healing begins with recognizing patterns instead of chasing individual complaints. For example, a person experiencing fatigue, digestive discomfort, and skin flare-ups might see three different specialists for each issue. In reality, all three symptoms can stem from the same underlying cause: chronic inflammation driven by gut imbalance. Addressing the gut restores energy, clears the skin, and stabilizes digestion all at once. This is the kind of connection that symptom-based approaches often miss.

Another limitation of symptom management is that it discourages personal agency. When health is reduced to prescriptions and test results, people stop trusting their own signals. They wait for an external authority to validate how they feel rather than learning to interpret their body's feedback. Restoring this connection is one of the most powerful outcomes of root-cause healing. It shifts the narrative from "What pill do I need?" to "What is my body asking for?" That change opens the door to real, lasting recovery.

Root-cause healing also respects that lifestyle factors — nutrition, sleep, stress, environment — often outweigh genetics in determining how you feel day to day. This is good news. It means you are not locked into a fixed outcome because of your DNA or family history. It means that small, consistent changes can dramatically alter your trajectory. It means your energy, mental clarity, and resilience are far more within your control than you have been led to believe.

This approach does not dismiss medicine or the value of doctors. It reframes their role. Acute care, surgery, and lifesaving interventions remain essential. But for the ongoing conditions that steal energy and quality of life, the most powerful solutions come from aligning your daily choices with your biology. That is what symptom-based medicine rarely provides — and what this protocol is designed to deliver.

Reclaiming your health starts by understanding these gaps in the system and choosing a new path. Once you see that symptoms are signals rather than enemies, you can work with your body instead of fighting against it. The rest of this book will guide you through identifying hidden stressors, supporting core systems like the gut and hormones, and building a practical reset that restores energy and reduces inflammation in a way that lasts.

The New Path: Root-Cause Healing in Real Life

When you understand that symptoms are signals, not random malfunctions, the way forward becomes clearer. Instead of silencing those signals with medication or ignoring them until they become unbearable, the goal is to identify what set them off in the first place. This is what root-cause healing offers: a chance to look beneath the surface and correct the conditions that create imbalance rather than endlessly chasing the effects.

Root-cause healing begins with a simple but often overlooked truth: the body is designed to heal. Every system — immune, digestive, hormonal, neurological — has built-in mechanisms for repair and balance. The problem isn't that these systems fail; it's that they are constantly overwhelmed by inputs they were never meant to handle. Over time, the body's repair signals are drowned out by processed foods, chronic stress, environmental toxins, and disrupted sleep. The solution is not to force healing but to remove what blocks it and supply what supports it.

How Root-Cause Healing Differs

Most approaches to wellness focus on adding things: more supplements, more superfoods, more biohacks. Root-cause healing often starts by subtracting. It asks: What is irritating your system? What is keeping your body stuck in defense mode? Only when those obstacles are cleared can supportive practices truly make a difference.

This perspective also views the body as an integrated whole. Your gut is not separate from your brain. Your hormones are not separate from your sleep. Energy, mood, and physical resilience are all connected through feedback loops. Addressing one system often improves others automatically. This is why someone who improves gut health might notice clearer thinking, better sleep, and fewer cravings — results that would never come from treating each symptom in isolation.

Practical Foundations of the Approach

In real life, root-cause healing is not about perfection. It is about creating conditions where the body can do what it is built to do. This involves four primary areas: reducing inflammatory triggers, supporting core systems like the gut and liver, stabilizing hormones and blood sugar, and restoring nervous system balance. None of these require extreme protocols or expensive interventions. They require clarity, consistency, and respect for how the body works.

One of the most encouraging truths about this approach is that small changes compound. Replacing one processed meal a day with whole foods can lower inflammation enough to improve energy. Swapping harsh cleaning products for non-toxic alternatives reduces daily chemical load in a way that supports hormonal balance. Prioritizing 30 extra minutes of quality sleep consistently can stabilize stress hormones better than many supplements. These are not dramatic actions, but their cumulative effect is profound.

Building this new path starts with observation. Many people live disconnected from their body's signals, dismissing fatigue or digestive discomfort as normal. Paying attention changes everything. When you begin to notice patterns — what foods leave you energized versus drained, how stress impacts your sleep, how certain environments affect your mood — you start to uncover the specific triggers unique to you. This awareness allows you to prioritize changes rather than attempting to overhaul your entire life at once.

Practical root-cause healing also depends on focusing your energy where it matters most. There is no shortage of advice online, but not all advice applies to every person. Instead of chasing the latest trend, the most effective approach is to target foundational areas. These include stabilizing blood sugar, improving gut health, reducing exposure to inflammatory foods and chemicals, and supporting restful sleep. Once these basics are in place, other layers of wellness — hormonal balance, mental clarity, resilience to stress — begin to improve naturally.

Consistency is more important than intensity. A single week of perfect eating will not undo years of imbalance, but steady improvements compounded over time can transform how you feel. This is why a structured plan is valuable: it removes guesswork and builds momentum. Knowing what to do each day prevents overwhelm and helps you recognize progress, even when changes feel subtle at first. The goal is not a quick fix but a shift toward habits that support your biology long term.

Another essential aspect of this path is flexibility. Your body changes with age, stress, and environment. What works for one phase of life may not work in another. Root-cause healing encourages curiosity rather than rigid rules. It teaches you to listen to feedback — energy levels, digestion, sleep quality — and adjust rather than forcing yourself to follow a protocol that no longer serves you. This adaptability is what makes the results sustainable.

The most profound impact of this approach often goes beyond physical health. When you begin to feel better, mental clarity improves. Mood stabilizes. Motivation returns. The fog lifts and life feels lighter, not because everything outside you has changed but because your internal state finally supports the life you want to live. This is where the true value lies: regaining the ability to fully show up in your work, your relationships, and your goals without constantly battling exhaustion.

The chapters ahead will walk you step by step through identifying triggers, understanding your body's responses, and building a protocol that fits your reality. By combining insight with practical actions, you'll create a foundation strong enough to carry you beyond short-term fixes into a way of living that restores energy and keeps inflammation under control for good.

Chapter 1: The Silent Saboteurs in Your Daily Life

Processed Foods and the Inflammatory Cascade

The foods we eat every day are not the same foods our bodies evolved to handle. In just a few decades, the modern diet has shifted dramatically toward processed, packaged options that are convenient but biologically disruptive. These foods often contain refined sugars, industrial oils, additives, and preservatives that the human body interprets as foreign. The result is not just weight gain or nutrient deficiency but a deeper response: chronic inflammation that affects nearly every system in the body.

Inflammation is the immune system's natural defense against harm. When you cut yourself or fight an infection, inflammation is what helps you heal. But when the immune system is constantly triggered by the foods you eat, it stops being protective and starts being destructive. Low-grade, persistent inflammation damages tissues, interferes with hormonal signaling, and disrupts energy production at the cellular level. This is why people can feel exhausted, achy, or foggy even without obvious illness.

What Makes Processed Foods So Problematic

Most processed foods are stripped of their natural structure and altered in ways that confuse the body. Refined carbohydrates like white flour and sugar cause rapid spikes in blood sugar, followed by crashes that stress the adrenal system and promote fat storage. Industrial seed oils, common in fried foods and packaged snacks, are high in omega-6 fatty acids, which are pro-inflammatory when consumed in excess. Artificial additives, preservatives, and flavor enhancers introduce compounds the body struggles to recognize, prompting an immune response similar to what would happen with a low-grade toxin.

This combination creates what researchers call an "inflammatory cascade." One trigger leads to another: unstable blood sugar raises cortisol, excess omega-6 oils disrupt cell membranes, and artificial chemicals burden the liver. Over time, this chain reaction feeds into the chronic fatigue, brain fog, and hormonal imbalances so many people face today.

The Subtlety of the Damage

One of the biggest challenges is that these effects are rarely immediate. Unlike food allergies, which can cause obvious reactions, the inflammatory response to processed foods is slower and quieter. Someone might eat fast food regularly without feeling ill right away, only to develop joint stiffness, digestive discomfort, or weight gain months or years later. Because the symptoms develop gradually, it's easy to dismiss them as unrelated or attribute them to aging.

Even so-called "healthy" processed foods can be problematic. Protein bars, diet shakes, and low-fat snacks often contain hidden sugars, artificial sweeteners, and emulsifiers that still disrupt gut health and fuel inflammation. Marketing claims like "low calorie" or "high protein" can mask the reality that these products are still highly engineered and far from the nutrient-dense foods the body thrives on.

The good news is that your body responds quickly when these inflammatory triggers are removed. Within days of shifting away from processed foods, many people notice less bloating, more stable energy, and even clearer thinking. These early improvements are not coincidences but signs that your immune system is no longer in a constant state of defense. As inflammation subsides, the body can redirect energy from fighting to repairing.

Reducing processed foods does not mean adopting perfection or never eating convenience items again. It begins with identifying the most common culprits in your own diet. For many, this means refined sugars, packaged snacks, fast food, and heavily processed grains. Replacing these with whole-food alternatives — fresh fruits, vegetables, quality proteins, healthy fats — provides the nutrients your body needs without the constant immune activation. The shift can feel dramatic at first, especially if your baseline has been years of refined foods, but the rewards build quickly.

An important part of this process is retraining taste preferences. Processed foods are engineered for hyper-palatability, meaning they are designed to override natural hunger and fullness cues. The high sugar, salt, and fat combinations light up the brain's reward centers, making whole foods seem bland by comparison. After a few weeks of consistent changes, taste buds adapt and natural flavors begin to feel satisfying again. This change is one of the clearest signs that the body is recalibrating toward balance.

As inflammation decreases, other systems begin to normalize. Blood sugar fluctuations become less severe, which stabilizes energy and mood. Hormonal communication improves, supporting better sleep and metabolism. Gut health recovers as irritants are removed, which in turn boosts immune function and mental clarity. Each small improvement feeds into the next, creating momentum toward lasting change rather than a temporary fix.

This process also highlights how deeply food impacts more than physical health. When energy improves and brain fog lifts, patience increases, focus sharpens, and stress feels easier to manage. These changes create a positive feedback loop where healthier choices feel rewarding rather than restrictive. Progress is no longer driven by willpower alone but by how good it feels to function at a higher level.

Understanding the inflammatory cascade caused by processed foods is about more than avoiding harm. It is about reclaiming the body's natural state of resilience. By removing the constant triggers and giving the body the resources it needs, you create space for healing that no supplement or shortcut can replicate. This is the foundation for the deeper work ahead: restoring gut balance, calming the nervous system, and building a sustainable protocol that supports vitality for years to come.

Toxins in Plastics, Water, and Household Products

Modern life surrounds us with conveniences that were unimaginable only a century ago. Plastic containers keep food fresh, cleaning products promise sparkling surfaces, and tap water arrives at the turn of a faucet. Yet hidden in these conveniences are chemicals that interact with the human body in ways most people never consider. They accumulate quietly, affecting hormones, immune function, and even the way the body stores fat. This is not about fear or avoidance of everything synthetic but about understanding where the greatest exposures come from and how they contribute to chronic inflammation.

Plastics and Endocrine Disruption

Plastics are among the most widely used materials on the planet. They also contain compounds such as bisphenol A (BPA) and phthalates, which have been shown to interfere with the endocrine system — the network of glands that regulate hormones. Even at very low levels, these substances can mimic or block hormones, particularly estrogen, leading to disruptions in metabolism, reproductive health, and mood. Heating plastic containers, storing fatty foods in plastic, or using disposable bottles repeatedly can increase the likelihood of these chemicals leaching into food and drink.

The challenge with endocrine disruptors is that their effects are cumulative and subtle. You may not feel an immediate reaction after drinking from a plastic bottle, but long-term exposure can contribute to weight gain, thyroid imbalances, or difficulty managing stress. Studies have linked these chemicals to increased inflammation and altered immune function, which explains why reducing exposure can lead to improvements in energy and mental clarity over time.

Water Quality Concerns

Water is essential for life, but not all water is equal. Municipal water supplies often contain chlorine, fluoride, and trace amounts of heavy metals or agricultural runoff. While these levels are typically regulated for safety, chronic low-level exposure can still burden the liver and kidneys, the organs responsible for detoxification. Contaminants such as lead, arsenic, or pesticide residues have been associated with hormonal disruptions, neurological effects, and immune stress, particularly in vulnerable populations like children and pregnant women.

Even bottled water is not always a solution. Many brands come from the same municipal sources, and the plastic containers themselves can contribute additional chemicals, especially if stored in heat. Understanding the local water supply, reviewing municipal water reports, and considering filtration options can significantly reduce these hidden exposures without creating unnecessary anxiety or expense.

Cleaning products, air fresheners, and personal care items are often overlooked as sources of chemical exposure. Many contain volatile organic compounds, synthetic fragrances, and preservatives that can irritate the respiratory system, disrupt hormones, or accumulate in body tissues. Fragrances labeled as "unscented" can still include masking agents that act as endocrine disruptors. Similarly, antibacterial soaps and surface sprays may rely on compounds like triclosan, which has been linked to altered thyroid function and increased resistance in bacteria.

Reducing exposure does not mean eliminating every cleaning product in your home. It means choosing options with fewer synthetic ingredients and using them strategically. Switching to fragrance-free products, opting for vinegar- or baking soda-based cleaners, and ensuring good ventilation when cleaning can significantly decrease inhalation of harmful compounds. For personal care, looking for short ingredient lists and avoiding products with unnecessary dyes or parabens can be a practical starting point.

Another important consideration is cumulative exposure. A single product may contain only trace amounts of potentially harmful chemicals, but most people use dozens of products daily. Toothpaste, shampoo, lotion, laundry detergent, dish soap, and deodorant all add up, creating a constant, low-level chemical load. This constant exposure can keep the immune system slightly activated, contributing to low-grade inflammation and making it harder for the body to reset.

One of the simplest ways to reduce this burden is to make changes gradually. Replacing every product at once can feel overwhelming and unnecessary. Instead, identify the items you use most often or that cover the largest surface areas of the body — such as body lotion or laundry detergent — and swap those first. Over time, this approach creates meaningful reductions without disrupting daily routines or requiring large upfront costs.

Water filtration and storage choices also play an important role in reducing exposure. Simple carbon filters can remove chlorine and some heavy metals, while more advanced reverse osmosis systems address a broader range of contaminants. For many households, a countertop or under-sink filter offers an affordable middle ground. Choosing glass or stainless steel containers for storage and drinking can also limit the intake of plastic-derived chemicals, especially when holding hot liquids or acidic foods.

The cumulative benefit of these changes is significant. When people reduce exposure to plastics, contaminants in water, and harsh household chemicals, they often notice improvements in energy, mood, and even skin health within weeks. These shifts happen because the body is no longer using so many resources to neutralize constant, low-level toxins. Freed from that burden, the immune system can focus on repair and resilience rather than constant defense.

This is not about living in fear of modern life. It is about making informed, intentional choices that lighten the toxic load on your body without adding stress. By understanding where the biggest exposures come from and addressing them step by step, you create an environment that supports healing rather than undermines it. This sets the stage for deeper work on gut health, hormonal balance, and nervous system regulation in the chapters to come.

Hidden Stressors: How Chronic Stress Fuels Physical Disease

Most people think of stress as something that happens only when life feels overwhelming — tight deadlines, financial worries, or relationship conflicts. But the body's stress response is far broader and more persistent than most realize. It reacts not just to emotional turmoil but to subtle physical triggers you might not even recognize: poor sleep, unstable blood sugar, environmental toxins, and even hidden gut imbalances. When these stressors become chronic, they quietly reshape biology in ways that fuel inflammation and disease.

The Physiology of Stress

Stress activates the hypothalamic-pituitary-adrenal (HPA) axis, a feedback loop that coordinates the release of cortisol and other stress hormones. In short bursts, this system is lifesaving. It mobilizes energy, sharpens focus, and prepares the body for immediate challenges. The problem arises when the stress signal never turns off. Instead of recovering, the body stays in a low-level state of alert. Cortisol remains elevated, blood sugar fluctuates, and inflammatory chemicals circulate continuously. Over time, this chronic activation erodes resilience rather than building it.

One of the first casualties of ongoing stress is sleep. Elevated cortisol at night interferes with melatonin production, making it difficult to fall asleep or stay asleep. Without deep restorative rest, the body cannot repair tissues, regulate hormones, or clear metabolic waste effectively. This sleep disruption then feeds back into the stress cycle, further elevating inflammation and fatigue.

Hidden Sources of Stress

Many stressors fly under the radar because they don't feel like "stress" in the conventional sense. Processed food spikes and crashes blood sugar, creating an internal stress response even if emotions feel calm. Constant notifications, noise pollution, or exposure to artificial light at night can all trigger low-level activation of the nervous system. Even unresolved gut issues, such as food sensitivities or microbiome imbalances, send danger signals through the vagus nerve, keeping the body in a defensive state without conscious awareness.

Modern work patterns compound these effects. Sitting for long periods, rarely going outside, and staying mentally "on" late into the evening deprive the body of the natural cues it relies on to regulate stress. The result is a mismatch between ancient biology and modern demands — the body thinks it is under siege even when nothing obvious is wrong.

Impact on Physical Health

Chronic stress is more than an emotional burden; it is a driver of physical disease. Persistently high cortisol raises blood pressure, disrupts thyroid function, and encourages fat storage around the abdomen. It suppresses immune defenses, leaving you more vulnerable to infections, yet paradoxically fuels autoimmune activity where the immune system attacks the body's own tissues. Inflammation rises, energy production falters, and neurotransmitters involved in mood and focus become imbalanced.

Over time, the body begins to adapt to this heightened stress state, but not in ways that serve long-term health. Cortisol levels may eventually swing from high to abnormally low as the adrenal system struggles to keep up, leaving you fatigued yet wired, unable to fully relax or find deep energy. This is why many people describe feeling tired during the day but restless at night, caught in a rhythm that no longer matches their natural circadian cycles.

The immune system also shifts under prolonged stress. Initially, it ramps up inflammation as a defensive measure, but chronic exposure can lead to immune dysregulation. This means the body may overreact to harmless substances, contributing to allergies or food sensitivities, or underreact to real threats, leaving you more susceptible to infections. Both extremes erode resilience and perpetuate the cycle of fatigue and dysfunction.

Hidden stress also alters the gut-brain connection. The digestive tract is lined with nerves and immune cells that communicate constantly with the brain. When stress is chronic, blood flow to the gut decreases, stomach acid production drops, and the microbiome shifts toward imbalances that favor inflammation. This can manifest as bloating, irregular bowel habits, and even mood changes, since many neurotransmitters are produced in the gut itself. Addressing these imbalances often improves not just digestion but energy, mental clarity, and emotional stability.

One of the most significant impacts of chronic stress is its effect on hormones beyond cortisol. The thyroid gland slows metabolism in response to ongoing stress, conserving energy as if preparing for famine. Sex hormones like estrogen, progesterone, and testosterone are also affected, which can disrupt menstrual cycles, lower libido, and contribute to mood swings. These shifts rarely happen in isolation; they create feedback loops that make weight loss harder, sleep less restorative, and emotional regulation more difficult.

Breaking this cycle begins with reducing the total load on the body rather than trying to eliminate stress entirely, which is unrealistic. Supporting the nervous system through better sleep, balanced blood sugar, regular movement, and intentional downtime gives the body a chance to recalibrate. Breathing techniques, mindfulness, and time in nature have been shown to shift the nervous system from a defensive state into one that promotes repair and recovery.

Making these adjustments does not have to be complicated. Small, consistent actions — pausing for deep breaths during the day, limiting stimulants, setting boundaries around work hours — signal safety to the body. Over weeks, these signals accumulate, lowering inflammation and allowing the immune and endocrine systems to reset. Many people are surprised at how quickly physical symptoms improve once the stress response is calmed, even without major dietary changes or supplements. The most important shift is understanding that stress is not just a mental experience but a physical one. When you learn to identify hidden stressors and respond proactively, you create an environment where healing can finally take root. This understanding prepares you to explore deeper elements of the protocol, where gut health, inflammation, and hormonal balance intersect to form the foundation of lasting vitality.

Chapter 2: Understanding Inflammation. The Real Root of Modern Illness

What Inflammation Actually Is (and Isn't)

Inflammation has become a buzzword in health conversations, but most people have only a vague sense of what it really means. It's often blamed for everything from fatigue to chronic disease, yet few understand that inflammation is not inherently bad. In fact, it is one of the body's most vital protective mechanisms. The real problem begins when this natural process becomes chronic, running in the background for months or years instead of turning off once healing is complete.

The Protective Side of Inflammation

When you cut your finger or catch a virus, inflammation is what allows your body to respond and repair. White blood cells rush to the injury or infection, releasing signaling molecules that increase blood flow and draw immune cells to the site. This process creates the familiar signs of redness, swelling, and warmth — all indicators that your body is actively healing. Without this acute response, even minor wounds or infections could become life-threatening.

This type of short-term inflammation is essential. It is the reason a sprained ankle eventually recovers and why a cold resolves after a few days. The system was designed for survival in environments where injuries and infections were the primary threats to health. The challenge is that modern life exposes us to different kinds of stressors: processed foods, environmental toxins, poor sleep, and constant mental strain. These do not cause visible swelling or pain, but they still trigger the immune system, keeping it in low-grade alert mode.

When Inflammation Turns Against You

Chronic inflammation is different. It is subtle, often silent, and systemic rather than localized. Instead of focusing on one injury or infection, the immune system remains activated throughout the body. Over time, this constant activity begins to damage healthy tissues. The process can disrupt hormones, slow metabolism, and even alter brain chemistry, which is why fatigue, brain fog, and mood changes are common symptoms.

The most frustrating aspect is that chronic inflammation does not always show up on standard medical tests until it has caused more significant harm. Many people are told their bloodwork is normal while they continue to feel unwell. By the time inflammation leads to a diagnosable condition — such as insulin resistance or autoimmune disease — it has often been simmering for years. Understanding this lag is key to taking action early, before symptoms escalate into something harder to reverse.

What Inflammation Isn't

Inflammation is not a disease by itself, nor is it an automatic sign of something "wrong" with your body. It is a communication tool — your immune system signaling that something needs attention. Labeling inflammation as the enemy oversimplifies the problem. The real goal is not to eliminate inflammation entirely but to regulate it. You want a system that can respond to real threats and then stand down when the threat is gone.

Chronic inflammation builds gradually, which is why it is often described as a "silent" problem. You may not notice it directly, but its effects are far-reaching. Energy becomes harder to sustain because inflammation interferes with mitochondria, the energy factories inside cells. Hormonal signals that control hunger, sleep, and stress response become less precise, leaving you tired but unable to rest, hungry even when you have eaten, or anxious without clear reason. The immune system, constantly activated, can begin misfiring, attacking the body's own tissues instead of protecting them.

This ongoing internal stress explains why so many seemingly unrelated symptoms cluster together. Someone might have joint stiffness, brain fog, and digestive discomfort at the same time. On the surface, these seem like separate issues, but beneath them is one unifying pattern: the immune system is stuck in an overactive state. Addressing each symptom in isolation misses the bigger picture. Calming the inflammatory response can improve all of these symptoms simultaneously because it addresses the common root.

The triggers for chronic inflammation are not always dramatic. Often they are found in daily habits and exposures: processed foods that spike blood sugar, low-level toxins in plastics or cleaning products, long-term sleep deprivation, and persistent psychological stress. These inputs may feel minor individually, but together they keep the immune system slightly activated at all times. Recognizing this cumulative effect is empowering because it means that small, consistent changes can significantly lower inflammation and restore balance.

One of the most important shifts in understanding is that inflammation is reversible. The body is constantly rebuilding and repairing, and when triggers are removed, healing begins surprisingly quickly. Blood sugar stabilizes within days, gut health starts improving in weeks, and even hormonal patterns can shift within months. The speed of this change depends on consistency rather than perfection. By steadily removing irritants and providing the body with nutrient-dense foods, restorative sleep, and stress management, the immune system gradually resets to a state of balance.

Understanding inflammation in this way also reframes health goals. Instead of chasing endless lab tests or extreme protocols, the focus becomes creating an environment where the body can regulate itself. This is less about fighting disease and more about supporting function. When the body is aligned with its natural design, energy, clarity, and resilience emerge as byproducts of that alignment.

This perspective forms the foundation for everything else in the protocol. Each strategy that follows — from improving gut health to balancing hormones and detoxifying the environment — is aimed at calming chronic inflammation and restoring the body's natural rhythms. Once this groundwork is laid, the body becomes far more responsive to healing, and the improvements extend beyond energy or mental clarity into every aspect of daily life.

How It Disrupts Hormones, Energy, and Immunity

When chronic inflammation lingers, it does more than cause discomfort. It rewires how the body communicates with itself. Hormones lose their balance, energy systems slow down, and immune defenses shift in unpredictable ways. These changes do not happen overnight. They build silently, often years before any obvious diagnosis appears. Understanding how this process unfolds explains why so many people feel tired, foggy, or unwell even when their medical tests come back "normal."

Hormonal Disruption

Hormones act like messengers, carrying instructions between organs and tissues. When inflammation is present, those messages become distorted. Cortisol, the body's primary stress hormone, is often the first to be affected. Initially, chronic inflammation drives cortisol levels higher as the body tries to contain the perceived threat. Over time, this constant demand can lead to cortisol dysregulation, leaving levels either too high or too low. The result is fatigue, mood swings, sleep problems, and a harder time coping with daily stress.

Inflammation also interferes with thyroid function. The thyroid gland controls metabolism, temperature regulation, and energy production. Inflammatory signals can slow the conversion of thyroid hormones into their active form, which leads to symptoms like weight gain, sluggishness, and cold intolerance even when thyroid tests appear within range. Many people who feel chronically tired may actually have inflammation suppressing thyroid activity rather than a primary thyroid disorder itself.

Sex hormones are not spared either. Estrogen, progesterone, and testosterone are sensitive to inflammatory stress. Women may experience irregular cycles, heightened premenstrual symptoms, or difficulty with fertility, while men may notice lower libido and energy. These imbalances are rarely random; they are part of the body's attempt to conserve energy and protect itself during perceived danger.

Energy Production Breakdown

Energy at the cellular level comes from mitochondria — tiny structures inside cells that convert food into usable fuel. Inflammation directly impairs mitochondrial function. It signals the body to shift energy toward immune activity rather than growth, repair, or mental focus. This is a survival mechanism in acute illness, but when prolonged, it leaves people feeling exhausted no matter how much they rest or eat.

This energy shift is why brain fog and physical fatigue often appear together. The brain is one of the most energy-demanding organs in the body. When mitochondria are compromised, concentration, memory, and motivation suffer. Physical performance declines as well, with muscles fatiguing faster and recovery from exercise taking longer.

The immune system's response to chronic inflammation is complex. At first, the heightened alertness provides extra defense against infections. Over time, however, this constant activity can lead to two opposite outcomes. In some people, immune defenses become suppressed, making them more vulnerable to colds, viruses, and slower wound healing. In others, the immune system becomes overly reactive, misidentifying the body's own tissues as threats. This is one of the ways autoimmune conditions begin, where the immune system attacks joints, the thyroid, or other organs. Both patterns stem from the same problem: the immune system has been operating in overdrive for too long.

The constant immune activation also diverts resources from daily maintenance. Repairing tissues, balancing neurotransmitters, and regulating hormones all take a back seat when the body is prioritizing defense. This is why someone with chronic inflammation can develop a wide range of symptoms that seem unrelated — digestive issues, skin problems, low energy, and mood swings — yet share the same underlying cause. Addressing inflammation at the root often leads to improvements across multiple areas because it frees up energy for the body to resume normal maintenance functions.

Another consequence is the feedback loop between inflammation and oxidative stress. As immune cells respond to perceived threats, they release molecules called free radicals. In controlled amounts, free radicals help fight infection and signal repair. When production is excessive, they damage cellular structures, including mitochondria. This damage further reduces energy production and perpetuates inflammation, creating a cycle that is difficult to break without deliberate intervention.

Breaking this cycle requires more than temporary symptom relief. It calls for a strategy that addresses multiple systems at once — calming immune overactivation, restoring mitochondrial efficiency, and rebalancing hormones. This is why protocols that target only one piece, like prescribing a stimulant for fatigue or a sedative for sleep, rarely create lasting change. The root issue persists unless the inflammatory burden itself is lowered.

Encouragingly, the body is designed to recalibrate once the pressure is removed. When inflammatory triggers are reduced, cortisol normalizes, thyroid function improves, and sex hormones stabilize. Mitochondria repair and multiply, boosting energy levels. The immune system shifts from constant defense to balanced vigilance, protecting against threats without harming the body's own tissues. These changes do not happen overnight, but they unfold steadily when the right conditions are in place.

Understanding these connections reframes how healing is approached. It is no longer about managing isolated symptoms or waiting for lab results to cross a threshold into "disease." It is about recognizing early warning signs and supporting the systems most affected by chronic inflammation before more serious conditions develop. By addressing hormones, energy, and immunity together, you create the foundation for sustained health rather than a cycle of temporary fixes.

The Three Stages of Chronic Inflammation and How to Reverse Them

Chronic inflammation is not something that appears overnight. It develops gradually, progressing through stages that reflect how deeply the immune system has become entrenched in defense mode. Recognizing these stages helps explain why some people experience only mild fatigue or occasional brain fog, while others struggle with widespread pain, hormonal chaos, or even autoimmune conditions. Understanding where you may be on this spectrum is essential for tailoring the steps needed to reverse the process and restore balance.

Stage One: Subtle Immune Activation

The first stage is often silent. It begins with minor triggers that the body perceives as threats — processed foods, poor sleep, or low-level toxins. At this point, the immune system is activated, but symptoms are minimal or nonspecific. You might notice slight dips in energy, occasional irritability, or mild digestive discomfort, but nothing severe enough to raise alarms. Standard blood tests rarely show abnormalities at this stage, which is why many people dismiss these early signs as stress or aging. Despite appearing harmless, this phase is critical. The immune system is already working harder than it should, using energy that would normally go toward repair and regeneration. If triggers persist, the body cannot reset, and low-grade inflammation becomes the new normal. Without intervention, this adaptation lays the groundwork for more serious imbalances.

Stage Two: Noticeable Dysregulation

As inflammation continues, the second stage emerges. Here, symptoms become more consistent and harder to ignore. Fatigue lingers even after rest, mental clarity decreases, and aches or digestive issues may appear regularly. Hormonal imbalances often surface during this phase, with disrupted sleep, irregular menstrual cycles, or sudden weight changes.

In this stage, the immune system begins affecting multiple systems at once. Blood sugar becomes harder to regulate, cortisol patterns flatten, and nutrient absorption declines. People in this phase often seek medical help, yet traditional tests may still appear normal or show only minor deviations. Without a clear diagnosis, they may be told everything is fine, reinforcing frustration and self-doubt.

Stage Three: Systemic Breakdown

At the final stage, chronic inflammation begins driving structural and functional damage across multiple systems. This is often where conditions like autoimmune disorders, metabolic syndrome, or persistent hormonal imbalances become diagnosable. The immune system, exhausted from constant activation, may start attacking healthy tissues or fail to recognize infections, creating a paradox of both overactivity and weakness.

People in this phase experience more pronounced and disruptive symptoms. Energy levels may fluctuate unpredictably, pain can become widespread, and mental clarity often deteriorates further. Mood swings, anxiety, or low motivation may appear as neurotransmitter production falters. The body is now operating in a state of conservation, prioritizing survival over growth and repair. While this stage can feel daunting, it is not irreversible. The body still retains its capacity to heal once the triggers are removed and supportive conditions are restored.

Reversing the Process

The good news is that healing can begin at any stage. The earlier inflammation is addressed, the faster recovery tends to be, but even long-standing issues can improve with consistent action. The first step is identifying and removing key triggers — processed foods, environmental toxins, and hidden stressors — that keep the immune system activated. Reducing this load allows inflammation to quiet down and shifts energy back toward repair.

Supporting foundational systems accelerates this reversal. Restoring gut health improves immune regulation and nutrient absorption. Stabilizing blood sugar through balanced meals reduces cortisol spikes and energy crashes. Prioritizing quality sleep and gentle movement calms the nervous system, creating an internal environment where healing can occur naturally. None of these steps are extreme; they are deliberate, steady adjustments that work with the body rather than against it.

In later stages, progress may unfold more gradually, but consistency leads to cumulative benefits. Energy begins to stabilize, mood lifts, and physical symptoms ease as inflammation recedes. Importantly, this process is not about perfection but about building sustainable habits that align with how the body is designed to function.

Looking Forward

Recognizing which stage you are in provides clarity and motivation. It helps you understand why certain symptoms appear together and why chasing quick fixes rarely works. By addressing the underlying inflammatory process, you move beyond symptom management toward true resilience. This shift is the foundation of the protocol that follows — a practical approach to restoring balance across systems and preventing the cycle from restarting.

As you move into the next chapters, the focus will turn to specific systems most affected by inflammation, beginning with the gut and its profound influence on energy, hormones, and immune function. This understanding sets the stage for practical strategies that transform not just symptoms, but the way you experience health in everyday life.

Chapter 3: Your Gut: The Forgotten Control Center

Microbiome 101: Why Gut Health Drives Everything

Your gut is more than just a tube that digests food. It is a living ecosystem, home to trillions of bacteria, fungi, and other microorganisms collectively known as the microbiome. This community outnumbers your human cells and influences almost every system in the body — from how you extract nutrients and regulate hormones to how you think, feel, and respond to stress. Understanding this ecosystem is essential for anyone trying to restore energy, reduce inflammation, or regain control over their health.

A Complex Ecosystem

The microbiome is like a rainforest: dense, diverse, and interconnected. Within this environment are hundreds of species, some beneficial, some neutral, and a few potentially harmful. When in balance, these microbes support digestion, protect against pathogens, and communicate directly with the immune system. They produce vitamins, break down fiber into anti-inflammatory compounds, and even influence neurotransmitters like serotonin and dopamine, which regulate mood and mental clarity.

Problems arise when this balance is disturbed — a state known as dysbiosis. Factors like processed foods, chronic stress, antibiotics, and environmental toxins can shift the composition of gut microbes, reducing diversity and allowing harmful strains to dominate. Dysbiosis doesn't always cause obvious digestive symptoms at first. It can manifest as fatigue, brain fog, skin issues, or hormonal imbalances, because the gut's influence extends far beyond digestion itself.

Gut-Immune Connection

Nearly 70 percent of the immune system resides in the gut. Specialized immune cells line the intestinal wall, constantly scanning for threats. This close relationship explains why gut health is central to managing inflammation. A balanced microbiome trains the immune system to respond appropriately, distinguishing between harmless foods and genuine dangers. When the gut barrier is compromised — a phenomenon often called "leaky gut" — undigested food particles and bacterial byproducts can enter the bloodstream, triggering widespread immune activation. This is one of the key drivers of chronic inflammation and its ripple effects throughout the body.

Gut-Brain Communication

The gut and brain are connected through the vagus nerve, forming what is often called the gut-brain axis. This two-way communication means that stress can alter gut function, and gut imbalances can, in turn, influence mood and cognition. Many neurotransmitters, including a large portion of serotonin, are produced in the gut. This is why improving gut health often leads to better mental clarity, reduced anxiety, and more stable mood — benefits that cannot be achieved through diet or mental health interventions alone if the gut is neglected.

Modern habits are one of the biggest threats to a balanced microbiome. Diets high in refined sugars and low in fiber starve beneficial bacteria and feed strains linked to inflammation. Antibiotics, while lifesaving when necessary, wipe out entire microbial populations, often without being fully rebuilt afterward. Chronic stress alters gut motility and reduces protective mucus layers, while lack of sleep disrupts the circadian rhythm of gut microbes themselves. Even exposure to environmental toxins and chemicals in food packaging can shift the microbial balance in subtle ways that accumulate over time.

When this balance is lost, the gut becomes more permeable and immune responses become exaggerated. The body begins reacting to everyday foods and internal signals as if they were threats. This is why people with gut imbalances often experience seemingly unrelated symptoms like joint pain, rashes, mood swings, or stubborn fatigue. These symptoms are not isolated issues but reflections of the same underlying imbalance within the gut-immune network.

Repairing this system starts with providing the right environment for beneficial microbes to thrive. Whole, unprocessed foods rich in natural fibers feed the good bacteria, allowing them to produce short-chain fatty acids that calm inflammation and strengthen the intestinal lining. Fermented foods such as sauerkraut, yogurt, and kefir introduce live cultures that help restore diversity. At the same time, reducing sugar, artificial additives, and heavily processed oils deprives harmful microbes of the conditions they rely on to dominate.

Equally important is giving the gut time to rest and recover. Consistent meal timing supports microbial rhythms, while adequate hydration and mindful eating reduce digestive stress. Addressing stress itself through relaxation practices, time in nature, or gentle movement allows the gut-brain axis to shift out of a defensive state, improving both digestion and mood. When these habits are applied steadily rather than as a temporary fix, they create conditions where gut diversity naturally reestablishes itself.

The most profound change comes when the gut's influence on the rest of the body becomes clear. As balance is restored, energy levels rise, mental fog lifts, and inflammation across the body begins to recede. Hormones regulate more predictably, immune responses calm, and cravings for processed foods often diminish without forced restriction. This is why gut health is often described as the foundation of overall wellness — because nearly every system depends on it functioning well. Strengthening the microbiome is not about perfection or following strict dietary rules. It is about understanding the central role this ecosystem plays in health and making daily choices that honor it. By supporting the gut first, you lay the groundwork for deeper healing in every other chapter of this protocol, from hormonal recovery to nervous system regulation. This understanding transforms gut care from a single task on a checklist to the central pillar of your long-term health strategy.

Leaky Gut, Food Sensitivities, and Immune Overload

The lining of your gut is designed to be both selective and protective. It allows nutrients and water to pass into the bloodstream while keeping bacteria, toxins, and undigested food particles contained within the digestive tract. When this barrier becomes compromised — a condition commonly referred to as "leaky gut" — substances that should remain in the gut begin to slip through. This breach places constant pressure on the immune system, which reacts as if the body is under attack, fueling widespread inflammation.

How the Gut Barrier Works

The intestinal lining is only one cell thick, yet it forms one of the body's most important defenses. Tight junctions between these cells act like gatekeepers, opening and closing to regulate what passes through. A healthy barrier keeps harmful substances out while allowing nutrients to be absorbed efficiently. This system works best when supported by a balanced microbiome, adequate nutrition, and minimal exposure to irritants.

When exposed to chronic stressors — processed foods, alcohol, infections, or toxins — these tight junctions loosen. The result is increased intestinal permeability, meaning particles that were never meant to enter the bloodstream can now do so. The immune system, detecting these foreign intruders, launches an inflammatory response. Over time, this response becomes chronic, contributing to symptoms that may seem unrelated to digestion, such as joint pain, headaches, or persistent fatigue.

Food Sensitivities and Their Role

Unlike immediate allergic reactions, food sensitivities are delayed and often subtle. They occur when the immune system overreacts to proteins in certain foods that have crossed the weakened gut barrier. Common triggers include gluten, dairy, soy, and sometimes even otherwise healthy foods like eggs or nuts. Because reactions can take hours or days to appear, it is difficult to connect symptoms directly to what was eaten.

These sensitivities add another layer of strain on the immune system. Each exposure reignites the inflammatory response, keeping the body in a cycle of defense rather than repair. People often find that removing these triggers for a period allows inflammation to calm and the gut lining to heal. This is why elimination diets, when done carefully and temporarily, can be a powerful tool for identifying hidden food triggers without resorting to guesswork or unproven testing.

As the immune system stays active against these constant intruders, it begins to shift into a state of overload. Instead of responding only to genuine threats, it reacts broadly and unpredictably. This heightened alert can make the body more sensitive to other irritants, including environmental chemicals, stress, and even changes in sleep or hormone patterns. What starts as a gut issue ripples outward, affecting energy, mood, and overall resilience.

This persistent immune activation also drains resources the body would normally use for repair and recovery. Nutrients are diverted toward defense rather than rebuilding tissues, balancing hormones, or producing neurotransmitters that support mental clarity. Over time, this depletion leaves people feeling depleted themselves — a sense of being tired but wired, inflamed yet uncertain why.

Reversing this cycle begins by calming the immune system through targeted changes to diet and lifestyle. Removing common inflammatory foods gives the gut lining space to heal, while introducing nutrient-dense, anti-inflammatory foods supports repair. This is not about long-term restriction but about creating a period of relief that allows the body to reset. Once balance is restored, many foods can be reintroduced successfully, confirming that the problem was never the food itself but the compromised barrier that misinterpreted it as harmful.

Healing also depends on rebuilding the gut lining. Nutrients like zinc, glutamine, and omega-3 fatty acids play critical roles in repairing intestinal cells and reducing inflammation. Fermented foods and prebiotic fibers encourage the growth of beneficial bacteria that protect the barrier and retrain the immune system to respond appropriately. Adequate sleep, stress reduction, and hydration are equally important, as these factors directly influence the integrity of the gut wall and the stability of immune responses.

The most transformative shift happens when symptoms in seemingly unrelated areas begin to resolve. Skin conditions clear, joint pain decreases, and energy stabilizes because the immune system is no longer in constant battle mode. Hormonal communication improves, cravings diminish, and mood becomes more balanced. These changes illustrate how deeply the gut influences the rest of the body and why addressing it can feel like lifting a weight off the entire system.

Understanding leaky gut and food sensitivities is not about fearing food or striving for perfection. It is about listening to the signals your body sends and removing the obstacles that keep it from thriving. With the right support and consistency, the immune system moves from constant defense to a state of balance, allowing the rest of the healing process to unfold naturally in the chapters ahead.

Repairing the Gut Wall: What Actually Works (and What Doesn't)

The gut lining is remarkably resilient. It regenerates rapidly, with most cells renewing every few days. Yet constant irritation from processed foods, stress, alcohol, and toxins can overwhelm this repair cycle, leaving the barrier in a chronic state of vulnerability. Restoring integrity to this lining is one of the most powerful ways to calm inflammation and improve overall health — but it requires understanding what truly supports healing and what commonly promoted "fixes" fail to deliver.

The Foundations of Gut Repair

Repairing the gut wall begins with removing what harms it. This might sound obvious, but it is often overlooked in favor of adding supplements or trendy protocols. If the irritants remain — refined sugars, inflammatory oils, excessive alcohol, chronic stress — the gut lining will continue to break down no matter how many supportive nutrients are introduced. Creating a clean slate by removing triggers is the first, non-negotiable step.

Once irritants are reduced, targeted nourishment becomes essential. The gut lining depends on certain nutrients to maintain tight junctions and repair damage. Glutamine, an amino acid, serves as a primary fuel source for intestinal cells and helps them rebuild. Zinc supports tissue repair and immune function, while omega-3 fatty acids reduce inflammatory signals that keep the gut in a reactive state. These nutrients are found naturally in foods like bone broth, fish, seeds, and leafy greens, and can be used strategically in supplement form when deficiencies are present.

The Role of Beneficial Bacteria

A thriving microbiome also plays a direct role in gut barrier integrity. Beneficial bacteria produce compounds called short-chain fatty acids, such as butyrate, that strengthen the intestinal lining and calm inflammation. When the microbiome is imbalanced, these protective compounds decrease, leaving the gut more susceptible to permeability.

Feeding beneficial microbes with prebiotic fibers — found in foods like onions, garlic, and asparagus — helps restore this protective effect. Introducing fermented foods can further diversify the microbiome, though these should be added gradually in sensitive individuals to avoid discomfort.

Myths and Missteps

Many gut-healing trends focus on restrictive diets or aggressive detox programs. While short-term elimination of problematic foods can help identify triggers, remaining on extremely limited diets for long periods often backfires. Over-restriction can reduce microbial diversity and deprive the gut of fibers needed to sustain beneficial bacteria. Similarly, overuse of probiotics without considering the broader diet can provide temporary relief but rarely addresses the root cause of gut barrier damage.

Another common misconception is that expensive cleanses or harsh detox products are necessary for healing. In reality, the liver and gut are already equipped with natural detoxification pathways that function best when supported with adequate hydration, balanced nutrition, and reduced exposure to irritants. Extreme protocols can create additional stress on the body and delay recovery rather than accelerate it.

Building a strong gut lining is less about dramatic interventions and more about creating the right environment for steady repair. Consistency matters more than intensity. Small daily habits compound: eating a variety of colorful vegetables, ensuring adequate protein for tissue repair, staying hydrated, and managing stress to prevent the nervous system from constantly signaling danger to the digestive tract. When these fundamentals are in place, the gut naturally begins to heal.

Stress management is often underestimated in this process. Psychological stress alone can increase gut permeability, even when diet is pristine. Practices like deep breathing, mindful eating, and regular movement help regulate the gut-brain axis, calming inflammatory signals sent through the vagus nerve. Without addressing stress, progress from dietary improvements alone is often limited.

Reintroduction is another critical phase often overlooked. After removing potential irritants and supporting repair, foods should be gradually reintroduced to assess tolerance. This prevents unnecessary long-term restrictions and helps identify which foods are genuine triggers versus which were only problematic because the gut was compromised. A structured reintroduction avoids fear around food and builds confidence in listening to the body's feedback.

It is also important to understand that supplements, while helpful, cannot replace foundational changes. Glutamine or probiotics may accelerate healing, but they are most effective when paired with whole foods and lifestyle shifts. Relying on supplements without addressing diet and environment often leads to temporary results rather than lasting resilience.

Healing the gut is not a linear journey. Some days will feel better than others, and occasional setbacks are normal. Progress is measured less by perfection and more by trends over time — clearer thinking, steadier energy, improved digestion, and reduced inflammatory symptoms. Tracking these subtle changes helps maintain motivation during the process and highlights how interconnected gut health is with every aspect of well-being.

Ultimately, repairing the gut wall is about restoring trust between the body and the foods it encounters daily. By removing triggers, nourishing tissues, supporting microbial balance, and respecting the role of stress and recovery, you create conditions where the gut can function as it was designed to. Once this barrier is restored, the benefits ripple outward, calming inflammation, supporting hormonal balance, and strengthening immune resilience — setting the stage for the deeper healing work that follows in later chapters.

Part II. Understanding the Body's Healing Systems

If the first part of this book revealed the hidden forces driving chronic inflammation and fatigue, this part shows how your body is built to recover. Beneath the layers of exhaustion and imbalance, there is a system designed to restore itself. Your hormones, gut, nervous system, and immune defenses are constantly communicating, adjusting, and repairing. The problem is not that these systems are broken — it is that they have been operating under conditions that prevent them from doing their job.

Modern life has disrupted the body's natural rhythms. Constant stress keeps cortisol high, processed foods disrupt the gut, and environmental toxins interfere with hormonal signals. These influences do not act in isolation; they overlap and compound each other, creating a cascade of effects that show up as fatigue, brain fog, weight gain, or anxiety. The key to lasting healing is not targeting one symptom at a time but understanding how these systems interact and restoring harmony between them.

This part of the book will take you inside these interconnected networks. You will see how the microbiome shapes immunity and mental clarity, how the thyroid and adrenal glands dictate energy levels, and how the nervous system controls the shift between fight-or-flight and rest-and-repair. Most importantly, you will learn how to support these systems with practical, sustainable changes rather than extreme measures or rigid protocols.

The goal here is clarity and empowerment. By understanding how your body is wired to heal, you gain the confidence to work with it rather than against it. This knowledge transforms small daily choices — what you eat, how you sleep, how you respond to stress — into powerful tools for recovery. With this foundation, the practical strategies in the next part of the book will make sense, feel manageable, and most importantly, deliver results that last.

Chapter 4: Hormonal Chaos and Energy Crashes

Cortisol, Thyroid, and the Stress-Weight Connection

Weight struggles are rarely just about calories in and calories out. Many people eat less, exercise more, and still feel stuck, their bodies holding onto weight despite their best efforts. One of the most overlooked reasons for this frustration lies in the interaction between cortisol and the thyroid — two key hormones deeply influenced by stress. Understanding how these systems work together, and how chronic stress disrupts them, reveals why weight and energy are so difficult to manage until underlying imbalances are addressed.

Cortisol: The Body's Survival Hormone

Cortisol is produced by the adrenal glands in response to stress. In short bursts, it is incredibly useful: it mobilizes energy, raises blood sugar to fuel quick action, and sharpens focus in moments of danger. The problem is that modern life keeps cortisol elevated far longer than the body was designed to handle. Constant notifications, deadlines, processed foods, and even lack of sleep can trigger this same survival response day after day.

When cortisol stays high, several changes occur. The body shifts energy away from digestion, reproduction, and long-term repair, prioritizing immediate survival. Blood sugar remains elevated to supply quick fuel, which leads to insulin spikes and, over time, increased fat storage — especially around the abdomen. Muscles may break down for energy, and cravings for high-calorie foods intensify as the body prepares for what it perceives as ongoing threat.

Thyroid Function Under Stress

The thyroid gland governs metabolism, energy production, and temperature regulation. It works closely with the adrenal glands, and when stress is chronic, thyroid function often slows. This happens because the body interprets constant stress as a signal to conserve energy. Levels of active thyroid hormone (T3) decrease, while the conversion of T4 to reverse T3 — an inactive form — increases. The result is sluggish metabolism, weight gain, fatigue, and difficulty maintaining body temperature.

This slowdown is often subtle enough that standard thyroid tests, which typically measure only TSH and sometimes T4, can appear normal. Many people are told their thyroid is fine even as they experience classic signs of underactive thyroid: weight that won't budge, cold hands and feet, thinning hair, and constant exhaustion. In reality, the issue lies not in thyroid hormone production but in its conversion and utilization — processes heavily influenced by inflammation and cortisol.

The Stress-Weight Cycle

When cortisol rises and thyroid function declines, a vicious cycle begins. High cortisol encourages fat storage, particularly visceral fat around the midsection. This fat tissue itself produces inflammatory chemicals that worsen hormonal imbalance. As inflammation increases, thyroid hormone conversion slows further, metabolism drops, and weight gain accelerates. The resulting frustration often leads people to restrict calories or overexercise, both of which can raise cortisol even more, deepening the cycle.

Restoring balance between cortisol and thyroid function starts with creating safety signals for the body. When the nervous system senses ongoing threat, it prioritizes survival over fat loss or hormonal harmony. Reducing stress through sleep, blood sugar stability, and relaxation practices tells the body it is safe to shift back toward repair and balanced metabolism. This shift is gradual but powerful, as it reverses the internal message that fuel must be conserved and fat must be stored.

Nutrition is central to this process. Meals built around whole foods with balanced protein, healthy fats, and fiber keep blood sugar steady and prevent the cortisol spikes caused by extreme highs and lows. Adequate calories are equally important. Undereating signals scarcity, driving cortisol higher and further suppressing thyroid function. Consistency in eating patterns helps retrain the body to trust that nourishment will be available, which allows stress hormones to normalize.

Supporting thyroid function also requires attention to specific nutrients. Selenium and zinc are critical for thyroid hormone conversion, while iodine supports hormone production in the first place. These are best obtained through a varied diet that includes seafood, nuts, seeds, and leafy greens rather than relying on isolated supplements unless a deficiency is confirmed. Anti-inflammatory foods, such as omega-3-rich fish and colorful vegetables, provide the antioxidants needed to protect thyroid tissue from further stress.

Movement plays a dual role in this process. Intense exercise can elevate cortisol temporarily, which is beneficial in short bursts but harmful if overdone. Gentle strength training, walking, and restorative practices like yoga or mobility work support metabolism without overstressing the adrenal system. The goal is not to push harder but to move in ways that energize rather than deplete. Over time, this recalibrates the stress response and improves energy availability for daily life.

Another overlooked factor is recovery. Quality sleep is where hormonal repair occurs. Without enough deep sleep, cortisol remains high, thyroid conversion stalls, and appetite-regulating hormones become disrupted. Prioritizing sleep hygiene — dimming lights in the evening, avoiding screens before bed, and maintaining consistent sleep and wake times — creates conditions for true recovery. These practices may seem small but have a profound impact on both weight and energy over time.

As cortisol levels stabilize and thyroid function improves, weight regulation often becomes easier without extreme diets or overtraining. People frequently notice that cravings diminish, energy levels rise, and their body composition changes even without dramatic calorie restriction. This shift comes from aligning with the body's natural rhythms rather than fighting them — a sustainable approach that builds resilience rather than depleting it further.

Addressing the stress-weight connection is not a quick fix but a reset of how the body perceives and responds to its environment. By focusing on calming the stress response, nourishing the thyroid, and supporting overall hormonal harmony, you create conditions where energy, metabolism, and mood can thrive. This foundation prepares the body for deeper healing and makes every other change — from gut repair to nervous system balance — far more effective in the chapters ahead.

Blood Sugar Swings and Why They Keep You Tired

Energy crashes are often blamed on stress, lack of sleep, or even aging, but one of the most common and overlooked culprits is unstable blood sugar. Many people live on a daily rollercoaster of highs and lows, where energy spikes briefly after a meal or snack, only to plummet a couple of hours later. This cycle creates fatigue, irritability, and cravings that feel impossible to control — and over time, it quietly contributes to inflammation and hormonal imbalance.

How Blood Sugar Works

Blood sugar, or glucose, is the body's primary source of energy. After you eat, carbohydrates are broken down into glucose, which enters the bloodstream. In response, the pancreas releases insulin, a hormone that helps shuttle glucose into cells where it can be used for fuel. Ideally, this process is smooth: blood sugar rises moderately after a meal and returns to baseline within a few hours.

The trouble begins when the system is constantly overloaded with refined carbohydrates and added sugars. White bread, pastries, sweetened drinks, and even many so-called "healthy" snacks cause rapid spikes in blood glucose. The body responds with a surge of insulin to bring levels back down. This drop is often more dramatic than needed, leaving blood sugar lower than optimal. The result is the familiar mid-morning or mid-afternoon slump, marked by fatigue, brain fog, and a sudden craving for more sugar or caffeine.

The Stress Connection

Blood sugar instability is not just a dietary issue — it is a stress issue. Each sharp rise and fall in glucose triggers the release of cortisol and adrenaline, hormones designed to mobilize energy in emergencies. When this happens multiple times a day, the body experiences it as chronic stress. Cortisol, in turn, disrupts thyroid function, encourages fat storage, and fuels inflammation, creating a cascade of effects far beyond momentary tiredness.

Over time, repeated spikes and crashes can lead to insulin resistance. In this state, cells stop responding effectively to insulin, forcing the body to produce more of it to manage blood sugar levels. Insulin resistance is a hallmark of metabolic dysfunction and a major contributor to weight gain, hormonal imbalance, and persistent fatigue. Even before it reaches this stage, the daily energy swings alone are enough to make life feel harder than it needs to be.

Stabilizing blood sugar begins with understanding the rhythm of your meals. When meals are skipped or spaced too far apart, the body compensates by raising cortisol to keep energy available. While this prevents a crash in the moment, it perpetuates the stress response and contributes to hormonal imbalance. Consistent meal timing — even if flexible — helps prevent these emergency signals and allows energy to remain steady throughout the day.

The composition of meals matters just as much as timing. Combining protein, healthy fats, and fiber with carbohydrates slows digestion and prevents sharp spikes in blood glucose. For example, pairing fruit with nuts or having whole grains alongside vegetables and quality protein provides steady energy rather than a quick burst followed by fatigue. Over time, this approach trains the body to use glucose more efficiently and reduces the frequency of cravings.

Choosing the right types of carbohydrates also plays a major role. Whole foods like sweet potatoes, legumes, and fruit provide natural sugars packaged with fiber and micronutrients, which help regulate their release into the bloodstream. In contrast, refined carbohydrates and sugary snacks provide immediate energy but leave you depleted just as quickly. Gradually shifting toward unprocessed options can feel surprisingly sustainable when paired with enough protein and fat to feel satisfied.

Lifestyle habits beyond food also influence blood sugar stability. Quality sleep improves insulin sensitivity, meaning the body can handle glucose more efficiently. Inadequate sleep, on the other hand, increases hunger hormones and drives cravings for quick energy, especially in the form of sugar or refined carbs. Gentle movement, like walking after meals, enhances glucose uptake by muscles and can dramatically reduce post-meal energy dips. Managing stress through breathing techniques or mindful breaks further supports balanced blood sugar by lowering cortisol and preventing unnecessary spikes.

Over time, these practices do more than prevent afternoon crashes. They create a foundation for hormonal balance, reduce inflammation, and help regulate weight without the extremes of restrictive dieting. Energy becomes more predictable, focus sharpens, and the emotional rollercoaster of cravings and irritability begins to level out. This stability is often one of the first signs that the body is shifting out of survival mode and into a state where deeper healing can happen.

Blood sugar balance is not about perfection or rigid rules. It is about building awareness of how food and habits affect your energy and making consistent choices that support stability. When you feel steady, everything else — from gut repair to thyroid support — becomes easier. This is the quiet power of balanced blood sugar: it transforms not only how you feel day to day but also how effectively your body can heal long term.

Restoring Hormonal Balance Without Gimmicks

Hormonal imbalance often feels overwhelming. Fatigue, mood swings, weight changes, and disrupted sleep can make it seem like the body is unpredictable and working against you. The health industry often capitalizes on this frustration, offering quick fixes — from detox teas to extreme protocols — that promise balance but rarely deliver lasting results. True hormonal restoration is slower and quieter. It happens when you address the environment your hormones operate in rather than chasing symptoms one at a time.

The Role of Foundational Habits

Hormones do not work in isolation. Cortisol, insulin, thyroid hormones, and sex hormones communicate constantly, adjusting to what you eat, how you sleep, and the stress you face daily. When one system is out of sync, others compensate, which is why symptoms often appear in clusters. Restoring balance begins by stabilizing the daily inputs your body receives: consistent meals, adequate rest, regular movement, and manageable stress. These are not glamorous solutions, but they create the conditions where the endocrine system can recalibrate on its own.

Nutrition That Supports Hormonal Repair

Food is one of the most powerful levers for hormonal health. Nutrient-dense meals provide the building blocks for hormone production and the antioxidants needed to protect glands from stress. Balanced macronutrients — adequate protein, healthy fats, and slow-digesting carbohydrates — prevent the blood sugar swings that drive cortisol spikes and estrogen imbalances. Micronutrients like magnesium, selenium, and zinc play key roles in thyroid function, reproductive hormone synthesis, and adrenal resilience. These are best obtained from whole foods: leafy greens, nuts, seeds, fish, and high-quality animal proteins form the foundation of a restorative diet.

Equally important is reducing what disrupts hormones. Highly processed foods, refined sugars, and industrial oils not only inflame the gut but also interfere with insulin signaling and estrogen metabolism. Alcohol, especially in excess, burdens the liver, which is critical for processing hormones. Removing or minimizing these stressors is as vital as adding nutrient-rich foods because it allows the body to redirect energy from defense toward repair.

Lifestyle Signals to the Endocrine System

Hormones respond to rhythms. Sleep-wake cycles, meal timing, and even exposure to light send powerful cues to the endocrine system about when to produce cortisol, melatonin, and other hormones. Poor sleep or irregular schedules confuse these signals, leading to cortisol spikes at night, low morning energy, and erratic appetite regulation. Establishing consistent routines — prioritizing sleep, natural light during the day, and winding down at night — helps reset these internal clocks and fosters natural hormonal balance without the need for extreme interventions.

Movement is another powerful signal for hormonal balance. Exercise improves insulin sensitivity, encourages proper thyroid hormone conversion, and stimulates the release of endorphins that stabilize mood. The key is matching intensity to your current capacity. Overexercising, especially with high-intensity training, can raise cortisol levels and worsen fatigue. Gentle strength training, walking, cycling, and mobility work provide the benefits of movement without overwhelming the adrenal system. Over time, as resilience builds, the body can handle and benefit from more demanding activity.

Recovery is equally essential and often overlooked. Hormonal recalibration happens during rest, not while pushing through constant stress. Deep sleep supports growth hormone release, tissue repair, and memory consolidation, while periods of relaxation during the day prevent cortisol from remaining elevated. Restorative practices like breathing exercises, time in nature, or simply unplugging from screens can reduce sympathetic nervous system activity and give the endocrine system space to reset.

An often-missed piece of hormonal healing is the role of the liver. The liver processes and clears hormones, including estrogen and cortisol.

When it is overloaded by toxins, alcohol, or poor diet, hormone metabolism slows, contributing to imbalances like estrogen dominance or sluggish cortisol clearance. Supporting the liver through hydration, high-fiber foods, cruciferous vegetables, and reduced exposure to environmental toxins can indirectly improve hormone balance without complicated detox plans.

As these foundational shifts take hold, symptoms begin to improve gradually but meaningfully. Cycles become more regular, energy stabilizes, and weight regulation feels less like an uphill battle. Mood swings ease as blood sugar and cortisol even out, and restorative sleep returns. These improvements reinforce each other — better sleep leads to better food choices, better nutrition supports hormone production, and balanced hormones make stress easier to handle.

What makes this approach sustainable is that it is not built on restriction or quick fixes. It focuses on creating an internal environment where hormones can self-regulate, rather than forcing short-term results through extreme measures. The body does not need gimmicks to heal; it needs consistent signals of safety, nourishment, and rhythm. When those are present, hormonal balance follows naturally.

This principle sets the stage for the next steps in the protocol: understanding how inflammation, gut health, and nervous system regulation interact with hormones to create either chronic stress or lasting vitality. By approaching hormones as part of this larger system, rather than isolated targets, you build a foundation for resilience that endures well beyond temporary fixes or seasonal health goals.

Chapter 5: The Hidden Role of Sleep and Circadian Rhythm

How Poor Sleep Fuels Inflammation and Weight Gain

Sleep is not just rest; it is an active process where the body repairs tissues, regulates hormones, and consolidates memory. When sleep is cut short or disrupted, these processes are interrupted, and the effects ripple through every system. Energy drops, cravings intensify, and inflammation rises, creating conditions that make weight loss and recovery far more difficult.

The Hormonal Impact of Sleep Loss

One of the most immediate effects of inadequate sleep is hormonal disruption. Cortisol, the primary stress hormone, should naturally decline in the evening and rise in the morning to help you wake refreshed. Poor sleep reverses this pattern, keeping cortisol elevated at night and blunting its rise in the morning. This mismatch drives morning fatigue, mid-day crashes, and evening restlessness, locking the body into a state of stress.

Leptin and ghrelin, hormones that regulate appetite, are also thrown off by sleep deprivation. Ghrelin, which stimulates hunger, rises, while leptin, which signals fullness, falls. This combination leads to stronger cravings for calorie-dense foods, especially sugar and refined carbs, as the body searches for quick energy to make up for lost rest. These cravings are not a lack of willpower; they are a predictable biological response to poor sleep.

Inflammation and Metabolic Slowdown

Sleep loss amplifies inflammation throughout the body. Studies show that even a single night of inadequate rest can raise inflammatory markers, and chronic sleep deprivation compounds this effect. This persistent immune activation contributes to joint pain, brain fog, and impaired recovery from exercise or stress. It also increases the risk of insulin resistance, where cells become less responsive to insulin's signal, leading to higher blood sugar and increased fat storage over time.

The thyroid is also affected. Sleep deprivation slows the conversion of thyroid hormones into their active form, leading to sluggish metabolism. This is one reason people who chronically undersleep often feel tired yet struggle to lose weight, even with calorie restriction or exercise. The body interprets lack of sleep as a signal to conserve energy and store fat, prioritizing survival over calorie burning.

Disrupted sleep also affects the body's internal clock, or circadian rhythm. This rhythm governs not only sleep and wake cycles but also digestion, hormone release, and even immune activity. When bedtime and wake times are inconsistent, or when screens and artificial light extend the day late into the evening, the body struggles to know when to rest and when to repair. Hormones like melatonin, which trigger deep sleep, are suppressed by blue light exposure, while cortisol remains elevated, keeping the nervous system on high alert. Over time, this mismatch leads to persistent fatigue and increased inflammation, even in people who think they are getting enough hours of sleep.

The nervous system plays a central role in this cycle. Poor sleep keeps the body in a sympathetic "fight-or-flight" state rather than a parasympathetic "rest-and-digest" mode. In this state, digestion slows, nutrient absorption declines, and recovery from daily stressors stalls. This imbalance can make even small stressors feel overwhelming, feeding into anxiety, emotional eating, and more restless nights. Addressing sleep quality, therefore, has ripple effects that extend far beyond energy levels.

Reversing the effects of poor sleep begins with restoring natural rhythms and supporting the body's ability to downshift into deep rest. Consistency is key. Going to bed and waking up at similar times each day anchors the circadian rhythm, making it easier to fall asleep and wake refreshed. Exposure to natural light in the morning helps signal to the brain that the day has begun, while dimming lights and reducing screen time in the evening tells the body it is safe to wind down.

Nutrition also influences sleep and inflammation. Stabilizing blood sugar throughout the day prevents cortisol surges that can interfere with nighttime rest. Including magnesium-rich foods like leafy greens and nuts supports relaxation, while avoiding heavy meals or excessive caffeine late in the day reduces digestive and hormonal disruptions. Small changes, like finishing the last meal two to three hours before bed, allow the body to focus on repair rather than digestion during sleep.

Quality sleep is not achieved through quick fixes but through steady alignment of daily habits with the body's natural biology. When these practices are in place, improvements can be dramatic. People often notice that cravings decrease, energy stabilizes, and weight loss happens more easily without major dietary restrictions. Inflammation markers decline, mood improves, and the nervous system becomes more resilient to everyday stressors.

Recognizing sleep as a cornerstone of healing reframes how recovery is approached. Rather than viewing rest as a luxury, it becomes one of the most powerful tools for resetting metabolism and calming inflammation. By protecting this process, the body regains its ability to regulate weight, hormones, and energy naturally, creating a foundation for the deeper protocols explored in the chapters ahead.

Resetting Your Circadian Clock for Healing

The circadian clock is the body's internal timekeeper. It regulates when you feel awake, when you feel sleepy, and even when your organs perform certain functions. Every cell has its own clock, but these are all coordinated by signals from light, food, and activity. When this rhythm is disrupted, everything from digestion to hormone release to immune function can fall out of sync, contributing to chronic inflammation, weight challenges, and persistent fatigue. Real healing begins when these rhythms are restored.

Why Circadian Rhythm Matters

The circadian rhythm does more than determine when you sleep and wake. It influences core biological processes like metabolism, cellular repair, and energy production. At night, during deep sleep, the brain clears metabolic waste and the body releases growth hormone for tissue repair. In the morning, cortisol rises naturally to help you wake and focus, while digestive enzymes and insulin sensitivity peak during daylight hours to optimize nutrient absorption.

When sleep and wake times are irregular, or when light exposure is misaligned with natural patterns, these processes lose their coordination. Cortisol may spike at night, making it hard to fall asleep, and stay low in the morning, leaving you groggy. Insulin sensitivity drops, increasing the likelihood of blood sugar swings. The immune system becomes confused, alternating between overactivity and suppression, which contributes to inflammation and weakens resilience over time.

Modern Habits and Disruption

Modern life constantly challenges the body's natural clock. Artificial lighting, late-night screen time, irregular work schedules, and caffeine use into the afternoon all send mixed signals to the brain. Food timing matters too. Eating late at night can shift circadian rhythms, forcing the body to process calories when it should be focusing on repair. Over time, these mismatches create a sense of always feeling "off" — tired at the wrong times, wired when you should be resting, and struggling with cravings or low energy throughout the day.

Small, consistent changes in how you manage light, food, and activity can reset this rhythm. Morning sunlight exposure helps signal the start of the day to your brain, anchoring cortisol patterns and boosting alertness. Reducing bright light at night, especially blue light from phones and computers, allows melatonin to rise naturally, preparing the body for restorative sleep. Aligning meals with daylight hours supports metabolism, while avoiding late-night snacking helps maintain hormonal balance overnight.

Reestablishing circadian balance works best when approached as a set of daily anchors rather than a rigid schedule. Consistency in key signals — light, food, movement, and rest — gradually retrains the body's internal clock to align with natural day-night cycles. This alignment improves not only sleep but also hormone regulation, energy stability, and inflammation control.

Morning exposure to natural light is one of the most effective ways to reset the clock. Stepping outside within an hour of waking, even for just ten to fifteen minutes, helps suppress residual melatonin and triggers a healthy rise in cortisol to promote alertness. This signal also strengthens the timing of evening melatonin release, making it easier to wind down at night. For people in darker climates or during winter, a light therapy box can be a helpful alternative, though natural sunlight remains ideal when possible.

Evening habits carry equal weight. Limiting exposure to bright and blue light in the hours before bed allows melatonin to rise naturally. Simple adjustments — dimming household lights, using warmer tones on devices, and creating a quiet pre-sleep routine — send powerful signals of safety to the nervous system. These cues prepare the body for rest, shifting it from a fight-or-flight state to one of repair and recovery.

Meal timing is another critical factor. Eating most calories during daylight hours aligns with the body's peak insulin sensitivity and digestive efficiency. Finishing the last meal two to three hours before bedtime reduces nighttime blood sugar fluctuations and supports deeper sleep.

Consistency matters more than perfection; even small shifts toward earlier, more predictable meals can make a noticeable difference in energy and metabolic health.

Movement throughout the day also reinforces circadian cues. Light activity in the morning and afternoon helps regulate cortisol patterns and improves insulin response, while avoiding strenuous exercise late in the evening prevents overstimulation of the nervous system. Gentle stretching or walking after dinner supports digestion without interfering with the body's transition toward rest.

As these practices take hold, most people begin noticing subtle improvements: falling asleep faster, waking more refreshed, and experiencing fewer energy crashes during the day. Over time, inflammation decreases as repair processes during sleep become more efficient, weight stabilizes more easily, and mental clarity improves. These benefits compound, making it easier to maintain other aspects of the healing protocol without constant reliance on willpower.

Restoring the circadian rhythm is less about strict rules and more about building a relationship with your body's natural signals. By aligning daily habits with this internal clock, you create an environment where healing unfolds organically. Once this rhythm is reestablished, every other system — from gut health to hormone balance — becomes more resilient, setting the stage for deeper recovery and sustained vitality.

Practical Sleep Protocols That Work in Real Life

Improving sleep is often presented as a matter of strict routines: perfect blackout curtains, no screens after sunset, a fixed bedtime every night. While these strategies help, they rarely fit the realities of modern life. Work, family obligations, and social demands make rigid routines unsustainable. What actually works is understanding the key drivers of quality sleep and building flexible habits that address them without adding stress.

Setting the Stage for Rest

Sleep quality is determined hours before bedtime. The way you manage light, food, and activity throughout the day directly influences how easily you fall asleep and how restorative that sleep is. Morning light exposure, consistent mealtimes, and regular movement all send cues to your body about when to feel alert and when to wind down. These daily anchors create a framework so that even if bedtime varies slightly, the body still recognizes when it is safe to rest.

Evening preparation begins with signaling to the nervous system that the day is ending. Dimming lights, lowering the volume of activities, and switching from stimulating tasks to calming ones are subtle but powerful cues. This transition allows cortisol to drop and melatonin to rise naturally, rather than forcing sleep in a state of alertness.

Managing Stimulants and Blood Sugar

Caffeine and sugar are two of the most common disruptors of sleep. Caffeine lingers in the body for hours, and even an afternoon cup can reduce deep sleep at night. Gradually shifting caffeine intake to earlier in the day helps avoid this interference without abrupt withdrawal. Blood sugar swings can also wake you at night as the body releases stress hormones to correct a drop in glucose. Balancing meals with protein, fat, and fiber reduces these fluctuations, leading to steadier energy during the day and fewer nighttime wake-ups.

Creating a Flexible Wind-Down Routine

A bedtime routine does not need to be elaborate, but it should be consistent in message: signaling safety and readiness for rest. This might include stretching, light reading, journaling, or simply dimming the lights and stepping away from screens. The goal is to cue the nervous system to shift from productivity to recovery. Flexibility matters; routines that feel like rigid rules often create stress when life inevitably disrupts them. Instead, think of it as a toolkit — a set of calming practices you can draw from depending on what the day allows.

Irregular schedules are one of the biggest challenges to consistent sleep. Shift work, parenting, or demanding jobs often make fixed bedtimes impossible. Instead of striving for perfect timing, aim for consistency where it matters most: the signals you send your body about when the day begins and ends. Anchoring wake-up routines, such as morning light exposure and movement, stabilizes circadian rhythm even when bedtime varies. On days off, keeping sleep and wake times within an hour of your usual schedule helps avoid the "jet lag" feeling that comes from drastic shifts.

Stress is another frequent disruptor, often showing up as difficulty falling asleep or waking in the early hours of the morning. Addressing stress during the day, rather than only at night, is key. Breathing exercises, short breaks away from screens, and mindful transitions between work and home environments reduce cumulative tension that otherwise spills into the night. At bedtime, simple relaxation techniques — slow breathing, progressive muscle relaxation, or guided meditation — help shift the nervous system into a state conducive to sleep.

Environmental factors also play a critical role. A quiet, cool, and dark space supports deeper sleep by minimizing external stimuli that can trigger micro-awakenings. Blackout curtains, white noise, and comfortable bedding can make a significant difference, especially in urban settings or shared living spaces. Even small adjustments, like reducing room temperature slightly or keeping electronics out of the bedroom, send strong cues to the body that this space is reserved for rest.

For those who wake frequently at night, identifying patterns can reveal hidden triggers. Blood sugar dips, late caffeine intake, or even dehydration can cause nighttime awakenings. A small evening snack with protein and complex carbohydrates may prevent drops in glucose that trigger stress hormones. Staying hydrated throughout the day, rather than drinking large amounts right before bed, reduces both dehydration and sleep disruptions from frequent trips to the bathroom.

The most effective sleep protocols are those that adapt to real life. Rather than seeking perfect conditions, focus on stacking small, consistent behaviors that collectively improve sleep quality. Over time, these habits reinforce one another: steadier energy leads to better food choices, calmer stress responses improve hormonal balance, and restorative sleep enhances resilience in every system of the body.

When sleep improves, healing accelerates. Inflammation decreases, cravings subside, and weight regulation becomes easier without extreme dieting or overexercising. Mental clarity returns, motivation rises, and the body becomes more responsive to all other aspects of the protocol. Sleep is not simply a pillar of health; it is the foundation that allows every other pillar to stand. Prioritizing it is not indulgent but essential — a decisive step toward restoring balance and creating lasting vitality.

Chapter 6: Nervous System Reset: Healing the Mind-Body Loop

The Biology of Chronic Stress and Trauma

Stress and trauma are often spoken about in emotional terms — worry, anxiety, fear — but their effects are rooted in biology. The body responds to every stressor, whether physical or psychological, through intricate hormonal and neurological pathways designed for survival. These pathways are protective in the short term but can become damaging when activated for too long. Understanding how this process unfolds helps explain why chronic stress and unresolved trauma contribute so powerfully to inflammation, fatigue, and disease.

The Stress Response: A Survival Mechanism

At the core of the stress response is the hypothalamic-pituitary-adrenal (HPA) axis. When the brain perceives a threat, the hypothalamus signals the pituitary gland, which in turn prompts the adrenal glands to release cortisol and adrenaline. These hormones mobilize energy, sharpen focus, and prepare the body for immediate action. Heart rate increases, blood sugar rises, and digestion slows so resources can be diverted toward dealing with the challenge.

This reaction is essential for survival in acute situations. The problem arises when the body remains in this heightened state without sufficient recovery. Modern stressors — financial strain, relationship conflict, constant notifications, and unresolved past trauma — rarely resolve quickly. The body interprets them as ongoing threats, keeping the HPA axis activated far beyond its intended timeframe.

From Acute Stress to Chronic Activation

When stress becomes chronic, cortisol levels often remain elevated for extended periods. Over time, this constant demand can lead to dysregulation, where cortisol becomes erratic — too high at some times of day, too low at others. This imbalance disrupts sleep, appetite, and energy, and can even contribute to mood disorders like anxiety and depression. It also drives inflammation by overactivating the immune system, which begins releasing signaling molecules that harm rather than heal.

Unresolved trauma adds another layer to this equation. Traumatic experiences can cause the nervous system to remain hypervigilant long after the event has passed. The amygdala, the brain's alarm center, becomes more sensitive, triggering stress responses to situations that may not be dangerous. This heightened reactivity can keep the body locked in fight-or-flight mode, draining resources and preventing the deep rest needed for recovery.

The Cost on the Body

Chronic activation of the stress response touches every major system. The digestive tract slows or becomes erratic, contributing to bloating, constipation, or diarrhea. Blood sugar regulation falters, increasing cravings and energy crashes. Hormonal systems adapt by prioritizing survival over reproduction, leading to irregular cycles, low libido, or fertility struggles. The immune system swings between overactivity, which can fuel autoimmune conditions, and suppression, which leaves the body more susceptible to infections.

Long-term stress and trauma also rewire neural pathways, especially those involved in emotion and decision-making. The prefrontal cortex, responsible for logic and impulse control, becomes less active, while the amygdala, which detects threats, becomes more dominant. This shift makes it harder to regulate emotions, concentrate, and respond calmly to everyday challenges. People often describe feeling "on edge" or "stuck in survival mode," even when nothing dangerous is happening in the moment.

This rewiring is not permanent. The brain is highly adaptable, a quality known as neuroplasticity. With the right conditions, neural pathways can be retrained, calming the amygdala's hypervigilance and strengthening circuits that promote resilience and a sense of safety. Practices like mindfulness, controlled breathing, and gradual exposure to safe experiences help reestablish balance in the nervous system, allowing the stress response to quiet rather than dominate.

Chronic activation also disrupts energy production at the cellular level. Mitochondria, the energy powerhouses of cells, work less efficiently under constant cortisol and inflammatory signaling. This contributes to fatigue that rest alone cannot fix. Cells shift from growth and repair toward defense, a pattern seen in people who feel depleted even after sleeping or taking time off. Supporting cellular health through nutrient-dense foods, stress reduction, and restorative movement gradually reverses this energy deficit.

The effects of stress and trauma extend to the immune system as well. In some people, prolonged stress suppresses immune defenses, leading to frequent infections or slow healing. In others, it triggers overactivity, where the immune system mistakenly attacks the body's own tissues. Both patterns stem from the same dysregulation — the immune system losing its ability to distinguish between real threats and harmless stimuli. This is why addressing stress biology often improves seemingly unrelated conditions, from autoimmune flares to seasonal allergies.

Healing requires addressing both the physical imprints of stress and the patterns of perception that keep the body on alert. This does not mean erasing memories or ignoring real challenges. It means teaching the nervous system that the danger has passed, so it no longer reacts to daily life as if it were a threat. Building safety through consistent routines, nourishing food, quality sleep, and supportive relationships creates the foundation for deeper therapeutic work if trauma is involved.

When these systems begin to regulate, people often notice changes that feel subtle but profound: calmer mornings, steadier energy, fewer digestive issues, and a clearer sense of focus. Over time, these improvements compound. The body conserves less energy for survival and redirects it toward repair and growth. This shift unlocks the body's innate ability to heal, transforming stress from an obstacle into an opportunity for resilience.

How to Calm the Overactive Stress Response

An overactive stress response keeps the body in a constant state of alert. Even minor challenges can feel overwhelming because the nervous system has lost its ability to distinguish real danger from daily life. This constant activation drives fatigue, inflammation, digestive issues, and hormonal imbalances, leaving many people feeling trapped in survival mode. Calming this response is not about eliminating stress entirely — that is impossible — but about teaching the body to return to balance more quickly and spend more time in a state of recovery.

Understanding the Sympathetic and Parasympathetic Systems

The stress response is controlled by two branches of the autonomic nervous system. The sympathetic branch activates fight-or-flight mode: heart rate rises, breathing quickens, and cortisol floods the bloodstream to prepare for action. The parasympathetic branch does the opposite, signaling rest, digestion, and repair. In a healthy system, these two states alternate fluidly, rising to meet challenges and calming down when the danger passes. Chronic stress disrupts this balance, leaving the sympathetic branch dominant.

Calming the stress response requires actively engaging the parasympathetic system. This can be done through consistent cues that signal safety to the body — deep breathing, gentle movement, nourishing foods, and predictable routines. Over time, these signals retrain the nervous system to respond more appropriately, reducing the constant background tension that fuels inflammation and exhaustion.

The Role of Breath

Breathing is one of the fastest ways to influence the nervous system. Shallow, rapid breathing signals danger, keeping the body in fight-or-flight mode. Slow, deep breathing does the opposite, activating the vagus nerve and shifting the body toward rest-and-digest. Practicing diaphragmatic breathing — where the belly rises on the inhale and falls on the exhale — even for a few minutes can quickly lower heart rate and calm the mind. Over time, making this type of breathing a habit can help prevent stress from escalating in the first place.

Why Predictability Matters

The nervous system thrives on predictability. Consistent sleep and meal times, daily routines, and clear boundaries around work and rest create a sense of safety that allows the body to let go of hypervigilance. This does not require rigid schedules; rather, it means reducing unpredictability where possible. Knowing when the next meal will be, when the day will wind down, and when rest is prioritized sends a powerful message to the brain that it is safe to relax.

Movement plays an equally important role in calming the stress response. Gentle physical activity helps discharge accumulated tension, regulate cortisol, and improve mood without overwhelming the body. Walking, stretching, or yoga performed at a comfortable pace signals safety to the nervous system. Unlike intense exercise, which can temporarily raise stress hormones, restorative movement supports balance by improving circulation and oxygen delivery while encouraging the body to release endorphins. Over time, consistent low-impact activity can transform how the nervous system reacts to daily challenges.

Nutrition can also either soothe or aggravate an overactive stress response. Meals built around whole foods, adequate protein, and healthy fats provide steady energy, avoiding the blood sugar spikes and crashes that trigger cortisol surges. Certain nutrients, like magnesium and omega-3 fatty acids, directly influence nervous system regulation and reduce inflammation associated with chronic stress. Minimizing stimulants such as caffeine and alcohol allows the body to reset more easily, preventing the heightened vigilance these substances often prolong.

Creating an environment that supports calm is just as important as internal practices. The brain is constantly scanning surroundings for cues of safety or danger. Clutter, constant noise, and overstimulation from screens can all subtly reinforce a state of alert. Simplifying the immediate environment — dimmer lights at night, organized spaces, and quiet moments without devices — provides ongoing reassurance to the nervous system that it is safe to relax.

Connection with others is one of the most powerful antidotes to chronic stress. Supportive relationships help regulate emotional responses through co-regulation — the natural calming effect that occurs when we feel safe with another person. Meaningful social interaction, whether with friends, family, or a trusted community, sends powerful safety signals that counteract the isolation and hypervigilance often seen in chronic stress states.

Finally, cultivating awareness of internal states is essential for long-term change. Practices like mindfulness or body scanning teach you to notice subtle signs of stress — tightening in the chest, shallow breathing, restless thoughts — before they escalate. Recognizing these signals early allows for gentle course corrections, like pausing to breathe deeply or stepping away from overstimulating situations. Over time, this builds a new default pattern: a nervous system that can rise to meet challenges when necessary but quickly returns to a state of calm once the challenge has passed.

Restoring balance to the stress response is not about eliminating life's pressures but about changing the body's relationship to them. With steady practice, the nervous system learns to interpret daily experiences as manageable rather than dangerous. This shift reduces inflammation, stabilizes hormones, and frees energy that was once locked in survival mode. It lays the foundation for every other aspect of healing, allowing the body to recover more deeply and respond more effectively to the changes explored in the rest of the protocol.

Simple Daily Practices to Rewire Safety and Healing

The nervous system learns through repetition. When it is used to scanning for danger, it will continue to do so automatically, even in safe situations. Healing requires teaching it a new pattern — one where safety becomes the default and the stress response activates only when truly necessary. This rewiring does not happen through a single breakthrough but through consistent, small practices that gradually reshape how the body interprets the world.

Why Daily Practice Matters

Safety cues must be experienced regularly for the nervous system to trust them. Occasional relaxation techniques may provide temporary relief, but lasting change comes from integrating calming signals throughout the day. Each time the body experiences safety — a deep breath, a grounding sensation, a supportive interaction — it updates its internal map, gradually lowering the baseline of hypervigilance. Over weeks and months, this shift becomes self-sustaining.

Breath as a Reset Tool

One of the simplest and most powerful ways to signal safety is through intentional breathing. Slow, steady breaths with longer exhales activate the parasympathetic system and tell the brain that the body is not in danger. This practice can be done anywhere — in traffic, at work, or during moments of anxiety — making it a reliable anchor in daily life. Over time, regular use of controlled breathing not only reduces acute stress but also increases overall resilience to future challenges.

Anchoring Through the Senses

Sensory grounding exercises help redirect attention from racing thoughts to the present moment. Feeling the texture of a chair beneath you, noticing sounds in the environment, or focusing on physical sensations like warmth or coolness provides immediate feedback that you are safe right now. These cues are particularly helpful for calming sudden spikes of anxiety or intrusive memories because they reorient the nervous system away from imagined threats and back to the current environment.

The Power of Predictable Routines

The nervous system thrives on patterns it can anticipate. Simple routines — morning light exposure, regular meals, consistent wind-down rituals at night — send repeated signals that the body can relax. This predictability reduces the constant scanning for danger and frees up energy for healing and repair. Importantly, routines do not need to be rigid; even loosely consistent patterns are enough to reinforce a sense of safety over time.

Movement reinforces feelings of safety by helping the body release tension accumulated throughout the day. Gentle forms of activity, such as walking, stretching, or light yoga, allow muscles to relax and signal that it is safe to exit fight-or-flight mode. Unlike high-intensity exercise, which can temporarily raise stress hormones, these practices support a gradual downshift toward calm. Done regularly, they help the nervous system associate movement with ease rather than strain.

Connection with others amplifies these effects. Supportive interactions — a conversation with a trusted friend, a hug, or simply sharing space with someone you feel safe around — activate pathways in the brain linked to social bonding and calm. This co-regulation is biologically powerful. Humans are wired to sense safety through others, and consistent, positive interactions can retrain the nervous system to expect safety instead of danger in everyday environments.

Reflection is another key component. Taking a few minutes each day to notice changes — improved energy, calmer reactions, or deeper sleep — reinforces progress and strengthens new patterns. Journaling, gratitude practices, or simply pausing to acknowledge improvements builds awareness of safety as it grows. This is not about forcing positivity but about retraining attention to notice what is stable and supportive rather than only what feels threatening.

Environmental cues play a subtle but significant role in maintaining this sense of safety. A calm, organized space reduces the background stress that clutter or chaos can create. Soft lighting in the evening, natural light during the day, and quiet spaces for rest help align the body with its natural rhythms. These cues may seem minor but collectively form a backdrop that supports every other practice in this protocol.

Over time, these daily practices compound. The nervous system becomes less reactive, cortisol levels stabilize, and the body spends more time in restorative states where healing can occur. People often notice gradual shifts: fewer energy crashes, less tension in the body, improved focus, and a deeper sense of calm even during stressful situations. These changes are signs that safety has been rewired — not as an abstract idea but as a lived, biological reality.

This foundation allows the rest of the healing protocol to work more effectively. Gut repair, hormonal balance, and inflammation reduction all progress faster when the stress response is no longer dominating energy and resources. By consistently signaling safety through breath, movement, connection, and environment, you teach your body to return to balance naturally. Over time, this becomes the new baseline — a state where healing is not just possible but sustainable.

Part III. The Reset and Practical Applications

Understanding why the body struggles is only half of the journey. The next step is learning how to apply this knowledge in ways that fit real life — not as a temporary program, but as a reset that rebuilds your foundation for the long term. This part of the book is about integration: taking the science of inflammation, hormones, gut health, and nervous system regulation and turning it into practical strategies you can live with every day.

Healing is not about perfection or following rigid rules. It is about shifting daily choices in a way that consistently sends your body signals of safety, nourishment, and balance. When these signals are repeated, the body begins to trust that it no longer needs to operate in survival mode. This trust allows energy to return, inflammation to calm, and systems like digestion and hormone regulation to function as they were designed to.

The focus here is on simplicity and sustainability. The practices outlined are designed to work even in busy, unpredictable lives. They emphasize building habits gradually rather than overhauling everything at once. Small, consistent changes compound over time, creating momentum without the burnout that comes from extreme approaches.

This part will guide you through key practical applications: how to design meals that stabilize blood sugar and support gut health, how to align sleep and activity with natural rhythms, and how to use simple nervous system practices to stay calm and focused in daily challenges. It will also show you how to adapt these strategies to different phases of healing — when energy is low, when stress levels spike, or when life throws curveballs that threaten your progress.

The goal is to equip you with tools that feel natural, not forced. By the time you finish this section, you will understand not just what to do but why each step matters, allowing you to make informed choices long after you have completed the initial reset. This is how temporary protocols become lifelong foundations for health and resilience.

Chapter 7: The 7-Day Reset Protocol

Phase 1: Eliminate and Detox (Without Extremes)

Detox has become one of the most misunderstood concepts in health. It is often marketed as juice cleanses, extreme fasts, or expensive supplement kits that promise rapid results but leave people depleted and frustrated. True detoxification looks very different. The body already has built-in systems for filtering and removing toxins — the liver, kidneys, lymphatic system, and even the skin. When these systems are supported rather than overloaded, they function efficiently without the need for extremes. This first phase of the reset focuses on removing what burdens these systems while providing the raw materials they need to do their job well.

Why Elimination Comes First

Healing begins with subtraction, not addition. Before adding new foods, supplements, or lifestyle practices, it is crucial to clear the constant irritants that drive inflammation and hormonal disruption. Processed foods, excessive sugar, refined oils, and artificial additives are common culprits. They keep the immune system in a heightened state of alert and interfere with digestion, blood sugar regulation, and energy balance. Eliminating these triggers allows the body to downshift from defense to repair, creating space for deeper healing in later phases of the protocol.

Equally important is identifying personal sensitivities that may not show up on standard tests. Foods like gluten, dairy, and soy are frequent irritants, though they are not inherently harmful to everyone. The elimination process is a structured way to temporarily remove common triggers, observe changes in symptoms, and later reintroduce them strategically. This is not about permanent restriction but about learning how your body responds so you can make informed choices long term.

Supporting Natural Detox Pathways

Once major irritants are removed, attention shifts to supporting the organs responsible for detoxification. The liver is central to this process, converting fat-soluble toxins into water-soluble forms that can be excreted through urine or bile. This requires nutrients like B vitamins, antioxidants, and amino acids found abundantly in whole foods such as leafy greens, cruciferous vegetables, berries, and high-quality proteins. Adequate hydration is equally critical; without enough water, the kidneys cannot flush toxins effectively, and the lymphatic system slows down.

Movement also plays a role. Gentle exercise improves circulation and lymphatic flow, helping the body transport waste products out of tissues. Sweating, whether from activity or time in a sauna, supports another route of elimination through the skin. These strategies are simple but powerful when combined with nutritional support, and they avoid the harshness of extreme detox programs that often deplete rather than replenish.

Implementing this phase is most effective when approached gradually rather than as an abrupt overhaul. Begin by removing obvious sources of processed foods — sugary drinks, packaged snacks, refined grains, and artificial additives. Replace them with whole food alternatives that are naturally satisfying and nutrient dense. This shift allows the palate and energy systems to adjust without the shock that often accompanies sudden restriction.

As irritants are removed, the body often begins signaling subtle improvements: clearer thinking, fewer energy crashes, and reduced bloating. These early changes are encouraging but should not be mistaken for completion. The goal is to create a calm internal environment, which may take weeks rather than days, especially if inflammation has been longstanding. During this period, paying attention to how you feel — sleep quality, digestion, mood — offers valuable feedback about what is working and where more support may be needed.

Hydration becomes especially important as detox pathways become more active. Aim for steady intake of water throughout the day rather than large amounts at once. Including mineral-rich fluids, such as diluted herbal teas or broths, helps replace electrolytes lost through increased elimination. Supporting hydration this way prevents the fatigue and headaches that sometimes occur when toxins are mobilized faster than they can be cleared.

Movement remains gentle during this stage. Activities like walking, stretching, or swimming encourage circulation and lymphatic flow without placing additional stress on the body. Intense exercise is best postponed until later phases, once energy and nutrient stores have been rebuilt. The focus now is on promoting flow rather than performance, allowing the body to prioritize repair.

An often-overlooked element of this phase is emotional detox. As physical stressors are removed, stored tension or stress patterns sometimes surface. Incorporating calming practices like breathing exercises, journaling, or quiet reflection helps the nervous system process these shifts. Emotional release is a sign of deeper healing, not a setback, and addressing it gently reinforces the overall reset.

Completion of the elimination and detox phase does not mean returning to old habits. The insight gained here forms the foundation for later stages. By learning which foods and lifestyle factors trigger inflammation, you gain clarity that guides sustainable choices. This phase is less about temporary cleansing and more about clearing the path for true repair — removing what no longer serves you so the body can use its resources to heal rather than defend.

Phase 2: Nourish and Repair (Foods, Habits, Environment)

Once the body has shed the constant irritants that fuel inflammation, the next phase is about rebuilding. Repair cannot happen in an environment of deprivation; it requires abundance — not in calories, but in nutrients, rest, and supportive habits. This stage is where energy begins to return, tissues start to heal, and resilience is built for the long term.

Focusing on Nutrient Density

The priority in this phase is providing the body with the raw materials it needs for repair. Nutrient-dense foods supply vitamins, minerals, antioxidants, and amino acids that support cell regeneration, hormone balance, and immune function. Colorful vegetables, fruits, high-quality proteins, and healthy fats become central. Rather than focusing on what to cut out, the emphasis shifts toward what to add: more variety, more quality, and more nourishment.

Cruciferous vegetables like broccoli and kale provide compounds that aid liver detox and hormone metabolism. Deeply colored berries offer antioxidants that reduce oxidative stress caused by inflammation. Wild fish, seeds, and nuts deliver omega-3 fatty acids, which are crucial for repairing cell membranes and calming the immune system. Together, these foods work synergistically to restore balance at a cellular level.

Rebuilding the Gut

The gut, often damaged by stress, poor diet, and toxins, begins to repair during this stage. Fiber from vegetables and whole foods feeds beneficial microbes, helping them produce short-chain fatty acids that strengthen the gut lining and regulate inflammation. Fermented foods like sauerkraut, kimchi, or kefir introduce live bacteria that support microbial diversity. These foods do not work instantly but gradually reestablish an ecosystem that supports digestion, nutrient absorption, and even mental health.

Hydration continues to play a key role, but now it shifts toward supporting cellular repair rather than just elimination. Adding mineral-rich options like coconut water, herbal infusions, or lightly salted broths helps restore electrolytes and supports energy production at a deeper level. Adequate hydration also keeps detox pathways functioning smoothly as the body repairs tissues and processes stored toxins released during the first phase.

Habits That Signal Repair

Healing is not only about food. The habits surrounding daily life send powerful signals about whether the body should prepare for survival or restoration. Consistent meal timing supports blood sugar balance, while mindful eating helps regulate appetite and improve digestion. Movement evolves from purely gentle activity to include strength-building exercises, which stimulate muscle repair and metabolic health without overwhelming the nervous system.

Environment is a crucial but often neglected element of healing. The spaces where you spend most of your time either reinforce repair or quietly keep you in survival mode. A cluttered, noisy, or chaotic environment signals the nervous system to stay on guard, while a clean and organized space encourages calm and focus. Simple changes like reducing unnecessary noise, improving natural light during the day, and creating a quiet wind-down space at night can have a measurable impact on stress levels and sleep quality.

Toxins in the home are another factor to consider. Cleaning products, plastics, and synthetic fragrances can add to the body's burden without you realizing it. Replacing harsh chemicals with gentler alternatives, improving ventilation, and using glass or stainless steel for food storage reduce daily exposure and allow the body to allocate resources toward repair rather than constant defense. These changes are not about perfection but about lowering the load wherever possible.

Social and emotional environments matter just as much as physical ones. Supportive relationships reinforce healing by reducing feelings of isolation and triggering calming responses in the nervous system.

Creating boundaries with sources of chronic stress — whether that means limiting exposure to constant news cycles, toxic conversations, or overcommitment — preserves energy for recovery. Surrounding yourself with people and activities that foster a sense of safety and connection accelerates the body's shift toward balance.

As this phase unfolds, energy typically becomes steadier and symptoms begin to ease. Improvements may show up first in digestion, sleep, or mental clarity, followed by more gradual shifts in weight regulation, skin health, and resilience to stress. These changes are signs that the body is reallocating resources from defense to growth, repairing tissues, and restoring balance at deeper levels.

Maintaining flexibility during this phase is important. Life will not always allow perfect meal timing, quiet environments, or uninterrupted routines, and that is acceptable. The aim is not flawless execution but consistency over time. Each nourishing meal, each restorative habit, and each supportive interaction contributes to cumulative healing, even if there are occasional missteps along the way.

By the end of this stage, the body is no longer merely free of irritants; it is actively rebuilding. Nutrient reserves are replenished, the gut is more resilient, and the nervous system is learning to trust a new baseline of safety. This foundation sets the stage for the next phase of the reset, where vitality is cultivated not just as recovery from stress but as a sustainable way of living.

Phase 3: Reintroduce and Personalize (Long-Term Success)

The final phase of the reset is where temporary changes evolve into a sustainable lifestyle. After reducing irritants and rebuilding nutrient reserves, the body is calmer, digestion is stronger, and energy is more stable. This is the ideal time to begin reintroducing foods and habits that were removed earlier — not to return to old patterns, but to learn which choices truly support you and which quietly work against you. This stage transforms the reset from a protocol into a personalized framework that can guide your health long term.

Why Reintroduction Matters

Elimination alone is not the goal. While removing potential triggers allows inflammation to settle, it does not reveal which foods or habits are truly problematic for you. Reintroduction provides clarity. By adding foods back one at a time and observing your body's responses, you identify patterns that lab tests often miss. This approach prevents unnecessary restriction and gives you freedom to enjoy a wider range of foods without guessing what might cause issues.

How to Reintroduce Safely

Reintroductions are most effective when done slowly and systematically. Start with one food at a time, ideally something nutrient dense that was removed during elimination. Eat a moderate amount of that food on the first day, then wait two to three days while monitoring for symptoms such as changes in digestion, energy, mood, or skin. If no reaction occurs, that food can likely be included regularly. If symptoms return, note the reaction and remove the food again for now.

This process requires patience but pays off in precision. Over time, you will build a clear map of what your body tolerates well and what triggers discomfort or inflammation. Many people discover that foods they assumed were problematic are actually fine, while others they considered harmless are the real culprits. This knowledge empowers confident choices rather than relying on restrictive rules.

Personalizing Beyond Food

Personalization extends beyond diet. The earlier phases also highlighted habits and environmental factors that influence your stress response and energy. This is the time to refine them. Some people thrive with early workouts, while others need gentle activity in the evening to unwind. Certain stress management techniques, like breathwork or journaling, resonate more strongly for some than others. Personalizing these routines ensures they fit your life rather than feeling like another checklist to maintain.

Long-term success depends on flexibility. The body's needs shift over time, influenced by seasons, stress levels, activity, and age. What works perfectly now may need adjustment later, and this is normal. Rather than clinging to a fixed set of rules, focus on learning how to read your body's signals. Energy levels, digestion, sleep quality, and mood are daily feedback systems that guide whether your current choices are supportive or need recalibration.

Maintenance also involves balancing structure with freedom. After weeks of intentional elimination and repair, it can be tempting to either stay overly strict or swing back to old habits. Both extremes miss the goal of this phase. The aim is not rigid control but an informed lifestyle — one that allows room for enjoyment while respecting what your body has taught you. Special meals, celebrations, and travel can be embraced without fear because you understand how to return to balance afterward. This stage is also about deepening awareness of non-food factors that affect health. Quality sleep, emotional regulation, meaningful connections, and time in nature are just as influential as nutrition. By this point, many people recognize that stress management is not optional; it is central to maintaining the benefits gained in earlier phases. Incorporating simple grounding practices — morning light exposure, regular movement, evening wind-downs — keeps the nervous system resilient even during busy or challenging periods.

Over time, the protocol becomes less about following steps and more about living with a new baseline of awareness. The body feels trustworthy again. Instead of second-guessing every symptom or chasing quick fixes, you approach health decisions with confidence, knowing how different foods and habits affect you personally. This confidence makes health sustainable because it no longer relies on strict programs or external rules but on your own informed intuition.

The greatest success of this phase is not just reduced inflammation or balanced hormones but the sense of agency it creates. You are no longer reacting to symptoms or chasing temporary solutions; you are proactively shaping an environment where your body can thrive. This shift transforms healing from a temporary goal into an ongoing process — one that supports not only physical well-being but also mental clarity, emotional stability, and overall quality of life.

When personalization becomes second nature, health stops feeling like a struggle and starts feeling like alignment. Every choice — what you eat, how you rest, how you respond to stress — reinforces the resilience you've built. From here, the path forward is not about perfection but about maintaining this alignment as life evolves, ensuring that your reset is not just a phase but the foundation for lasting vitality.

Chapter 8: Whole Foods vs. "Frankenstein" Foods

Identifying Real Food vs. Ultra-Processed Food

Food is the foundation of any healing protocol, yet modern food systems make it increasingly difficult to distinguish what truly nourishes the body from what quietly drives inflammation and imbalance. Labels often highlight protein or vitamins while concealing additives, refined oils, and sugars that overwhelm the gut and stress hormonal systems. Learning to tell real food from ultra-processed products is a skill that transforms not only how you eat but how you feel every day.

What Defines Real Food

Real food is minimally altered from its natural state. Fruits, vegetables, whole grains, nuts, seeds, meat, fish, and eggs contain nutrients in the balance nature intended. These foods require little interpretation — an apple looks like an apple, and a piece of salmon is clearly a piece of salmon. While some processing, like freezing or chopping, makes real food more accessible, the nutritional integrity remains intact. The body recognizes these foods and knows how to use them for energy, repair, and immune support.

Real food also provides complex combinations of nutrients that work together in ways supplements cannot replicate. The antioxidants in berries, for example, come packaged with fiber and plant compounds that support gut health and blood sugar balance. The amino acids in eggs are paired with healthy fats and choline, a nutrient essential for brain function. This natural synergy is why whole foods form the backbone of every healing approach.

Understanding Ultra-Processed Foods

Ultra-processed foods, by contrast, are products engineered to be hyper-palatable, shelf-stable, and convenient. They often begin as refined grains or oils stripped of fiber and nutrients, then recombined with sugars, flavorings, and additives to create something far removed from its original source. These foods are designed to trigger cravings, override natural satiety signals, and encourage overeating.

Common examples include packaged snack foods, sugary cereals, frozen meals, soft drinks, and fast-food items. Even foods marketed as "healthy" — protein bars, flavored yogurts, low-fat snacks — often fall into this category because of their reliance on additives, artificial sweeteners, or refined ingredients. The problem is not occasional enjoyment but the cumulative effect of relying on these products daily, which can disrupt blood sugar, inflame the gut, and keep the body in a low-level stress state.

Hidden Ingredients That Matter

Ultra-processed foods are not always obvious. Many appear wholesome at first glance, with labels boasting whole grains, added vitamins, or natural flavors. The key lies in reading ingredient lists rather than front-of-package claims. Long lists with unfamiliar names, especially preservatives, emulsifiers, and artificial sweeteners, often indicate heavy processing. Refined seed oils like soybean, canola, or sunflower oil, frequently used in packaged snacks and restaurant foods, are another sign; they are cheap, highly processed, and prone to oxidation, which fuels inflammation.

Learning to recognize real food becomes easier when focusing on simplicity. Foods with single or few ingredients are generally more reliable than those with long ingredient lists. Fresh produce, unflavored dairy, whole cuts of meat, and grains in their intact form require little decoding. When shopping, aim to fill most of the cart from the perimeter of the store, where fresh foods are usually located, rather than the inner aisles dominated by boxed and packaged items.

Cooking at home is one of the most effective ways to ensure meals remain centered on real food. Preparing meals from scratch allows you to control ingredients and avoid unnecessary additives. Even basic cooking techniques — roasting vegetables, simmering broths, or preparing simple proteins — create nutrient-dense meals without relying on prepackaged shortcuts. Over time, taste preferences often shift toward these foods as the palate adjusts away from the hyper-flavors of processed products.

Transitioning away from ultra-processed foods does not have to be abrupt or overwhelming. Replacing them gradually with real-food alternatives helps the body adapt and prevents feelings of restriction. Swapping sugary breakfast cereals for oatmeal with fruit, replacing packaged snacks with nuts or fresh produce, and choosing water or herbal teas over sweetened beverages are small shifts that add up significantly over weeks and months.

Awareness also helps break the emotional and habitual ties to processed foods. Many of these products are designed to trigger reward pathways in the brain, creating cycles of craving and overconsumption. By understanding this, you can approach them with curiosity rather than guilt, noticing how they affect mood, energy, and digestion compared to real foods. This awareness turns choices into conscious decisions rather than automatic habits.

As real food becomes the foundation of daily meals, energy levels often stabilize, cravings diminish, and inflammation gradually reduces. These changes are not just physical but mental; clearer thinking, steadier moods, and improved focus often follow. The body thrives when it is nourished with what it recognizes and can use efficiently. Ultra-processed foods, while convenient, keep the body in a constant state of compensation, always trying to balance blood sugar swings, manage additives, and repair low-level damage.

Identifying and choosing real food is not about perfection or never enjoying treats again. It is about shifting the default toward nourishment, so occasional indulgences do not derail progress. Over time, this approach becomes intuitive. Grocery trips are simpler, cravings for hyper-processed products fade, and meals feel more satisfying. This is not a temporary diet but a foundation for long-term resilience — one that supports every other aspect of the reset and ensures results are sustainable well beyond the initial protocol.

Anti-Inflammatory Foods and Their Science-Backed Benefits

Chronic inflammation underlies many modern health problems — from fatigue and joint pain to hormonal imbalance and digestive issues. While inflammation is the body's natural defense mechanism against injury or infection, it becomes harmful when it persists at low levels for months or years. One of the most powerful ways to calm this process is through food. Anti-inflammatory foods do not just reduce symptoms; they actively repair tissues, balance the immune system, and support long-term resilience.

The Role of Nutrients in Inflammation Control

Anti-inflammatory foods work by delivering compounds that neutralize oxidative stress and regulate immune signaling. Polyphenols, omega-3 fatty acids, vitamins, and minerals all play unique roles. For example, vitamin C helps reduce free radical damage, while magnesium lowers stress responses that can fuel inflammation. When consumed consistently, these nutrients shift the body toward a state of repair rather than defense.

Whole foods also influence the gut microbiome, which in turn regulates immune activity. Fiber-rich fruits and vegetables feed beneficial bacteria, leading to the production of short-chain fatty acids that strengthen the gut lining and prevent inflammatory molecules from entering the bloodstream. This connection between gut health and inflammation is why diets rich in real, plant-based foods consistently show benefits across so many chronic conditions.

Key Anti-Inflammatory Foods

Fatty fish like salmon, sardines, and mackerel are among the best sources of omega-3 fatty acids, which directly lower inflammatory markers such as C-reactive protein. Leafy greens — spinach, kale, arugula — provide magnesium and antioxidants that support detoxification and hormone balance. Berries are packed with anthocyanins, compounds that reduce oxidative stress and improve vascular health. Nuts and seeds, especially walnuts and flaxseeds, supply both healthy fats and minerals crucial for calming immune responses.

Spices also play a notable role. Turmeric contains curcumin, a compound shown to inhibit inflammatory pathways at the cellular level. Ginger supports digestion and reduces inflammatory signaling linked to muscle soreness and joint pain. These foods are potent yet safe, offering benefits without the side effects of many pharmaceutical anti-inflammatories when incorporated into a balanced diet.

Balancing Blood Sugar and Hormones

Anti-inflammatory eating is not only about individual foods but also about stabilizing blood sugar and supporting hormonal health. Constant blood sugar spikes trigger inflammatory cascades and stress hormone release. Combining protein, fiber, and healthy fats with carbohydrates slows digestion, preventing these spikes and supporting steady energy. Over time, this balance reduces strain on the adrenal and thyroid systems, which are often disrupted in chronic illness.

Incorporating anti-inflammatory foods consistently is most effective when approached as part of everyday meals rather than occasional additions. A plate built around vegetables, quality protein, and healthy fats naturally provides the compounds that calm inflammation without requiring complicated tracking. For example, pairing salmon with leafy greens and roasted sweet potatoes delivers omega-3s, antioxidants, and fiber in one balanced meal. Adding herbs and spices like turmeric or rosemary not only enhances flavor but provides additional phytonutrients that support cellular repair.

The benefits of these foods are cumulative. While a single meal will not transform inflammation overnight, regular exposure to these compounds steadily shifts the body's baseline. People often notice subtle changes first — improved energy, clearer thinking, fewer afternoon crashes. Over weeks, more tangible improvements emerge, such as reduced joint discomfort, better digestion, and more stable moods. These changes signal that inflammation is no longer dominating daily function and that the body's natural repair processes are regaining control.

Individual response to anti-inflammatory foods can vary, and personalization is important. Some people thrive on higher amounts of fatty fish, while others benefit most from abundant leafy greens or fermented foods. Paying attention to how different meals affect energy, digestion, and mood provides guidance for tailoring the approach. Keeping variety high ensures a broader range of nutrients and prevents reliance on any single food or supplement.

Equally critical is the quality of these foods. Organic or responsibly grown produce reduces exposure to pesticides that can burden detox pathways. Wild or sustainably sourced fish avoids contaminants found in some farmed varieties. Nuts and seeds are best consumed fresh rather than heavily processed into sweetened bars or flavored snacks. Choosing quality where possible magnifies the benefits of an anti-inflammatory diet without requiring perfection in every purchase.

Beyond reducing inflammation, this way of eating naturally supports other aspects of healing addressed in the reset. Steady blood sugar, improved gut health, and better hormone balance all arise from the same nutrient-dense, whole-food patterns. Rather than being a temporary protocol, it becomes a sustainable foundation that adapts to changing needs over time. This is why anti-inflammatory eating is not just a phase but a cornerstone of long-term vitality — a way of living that protects against chronic illness and nurtures resilience at every stage of life.

When Supplements Help — And When They're a Waste of Money

Supplements can be powerful tools for healing, but they are often misunderstood and overused. The wellness industry markets pills and powders as quick fixes, promising energy, detox, or fat loss without addressing the underlying causes of imbalance. This leads many people to spend significant money on products that deliver little benefit, or worse, add unnecessary stress to the body. Understanding when supplements are genuinely helpful — and when they are unnecessary — prevents wasted effort and supports a more targeted approach to health.

Why Food Comes First

Whole foods provide nutrients in a complex matrix that supplements cannot replicate. Vitamins and minerals in real foods come with co-factors — plant compounds, enzymes, and fibers — that enhance absorption and work together in ways isolated nutrients cannot. For example, vitamin C in citrus fruits pairs with bioflavonoids that boost its antioxidant effects. Calcium in leafy greens comes with magnesium and vitamin K, which are essential for proper utilization in bones and tissues. Supplements can fill gaps but should never replace a nutrient-rich diet. If the foundation of nutrition is lacking, even high-quality supplements cannot fully correct the imbalance. This is why the earlier phases of the reset focus on improving diet first; supplementation is most effective once the body is already supported by real food.

Situations Where Supplements Can Help

There are times when supplementation provides a clear benefit. Nutrient deficiencies, confirmed through testing or symptoms, are the most straightforward case. Vitamin D is a common example; many people have insufficient levels due to limited sun exposure, and supplementing can restore balance and improve immune and bone health. Omega-3 fatty acids, often lacking in modern diets, can also be helpful when fish intake is low.

95

Targeted supplementation can also support healing during periods of stress or increased demand. Magnesium can calm the nervous system and improve sleep, particularly for those with high stress levels. Probiotics may assist gut repair when used alongside dietary changes, especially after antibiotics or digestive illnesses. These tools are most effective when chosen for a specific purpose, rather than as a blanket approach.

Supplements often become wasteful when used as a shortcut in place of foundational habits. No capsule can replace consistent sleep, balanced meals, or stress management. Multivitamins, for example, are widely marketed as insurance against poor diets, yet research shows they rarely improve outcomes for otherwise healthy individuals eating varied foods. The same is true for trendy detox blends, fat burners, or "miracle" powders that promise energy and rapid weight loss; they rarely deliver measurable results and can sometimes strain the liver or digestive system. Quality is another concern. The supplement industry is loosely regulated, meaning products can vary widely in purity and potency. Some contain fillers or additives that do little for health, while others include doses far higher or lower than stated on the label. Choosing third-party tested products and focusing on reputable brands minimizes these risks. It is also worth questioning whether a supplement's marketing claims align with solid evidence rather than testimonials or hype.

Cost is a factor many people overlook. A handful of targeted, well-chosen supplements can be valuable, but stacking dozens of products quickly becomes expensive without providing additional benefit. The most effective strategy is minimal and intentional: identify clear needs through testing or careful observation, choose high-quality products that address those needs, and reevaluate regularly rather than taking the same pills indefinitely.

A practical approach involves prioritizing nutrients most likely to be deficient or difficult to obtain from diet alone. Vitamin D, omega-3 fatty acids, magnesium, and occasionally probiotics or B vitamins are among the most common candidates. Beyond these, most people can meet their needs through whole foods, provided their diet is diverse and nutrient dense. Working with a qualified practitioner can help determine whether supplementation is necessary, avoiding both underuse and excess.

Long-term reliance on unnecessary supplements can sometimes signal a deeper issue: mistrust in the body's ability to heal or a belief that more is always better. Shifting the focus toward nourishment, movement, rest, and emotional balance creates the conditions where fewer supplements are needed at all. When the body receives consistent signals of safety and adequate nutrition, it often corrects imbalances naturally, reducing the need for constant external input.

Ultimately, supplements should enhance rather than replace the fundamentals of health. They are tools, not crutches. When chosen intentionally and used in the context of a nutrient-rich lifestyle, they can accelerate recovery and support resilience. When used indiscriminately or as a substitute for real food and rest, they become little more than an expensive distraction. The key lies in discernment: knowing what is essential, what is optional, and what is unnecessary for your unique body and goals.

Chapter 9: Movement That Heals Instead of Hurts

Why Exercise Can Backfire in an Inflamed Body

Exercise is often seen as a universal solution to health problems — a way to lose weight, boost energy, and strengthen the body. While movement is essential for long-term vitality, pushing too hard at the wrong time can make inflammation worse rather than better. For individuals already dealing with fatigue, joint pain, or hormonal imbalances, high-intensity or excessive exercise may create additional stress the body is not equipped to handle. Understanding this paradox is key to designing a movement plan that heals instead of harms.

The Stress Response and Exercise

Physical activity is a controlled form of stress. During exercise, cortisol and adrenaline rise to mobilize energy and fuel muscles. In a healthy body, this response is temporary and followed by recovery, where inflammation subsides, tissues repair, and fitness improves. In a body already burdened by chronic stress or inflammation, however, this recovery window is compromised. Cortisol may remain elevated long after the workout, blood sugar regulation may falter, and immune activity may become more erratic rather than more balanced.

This is why some people experience worsening fatigue, poor sleep, or even weight gain despite exercising regularly. Instead of building resilience, their workouts deepen the stress cycle — layering physical strain on top of emotional and environmental pressures. Without adequate recovery, the benefits of exercise are lost, and symptoms of overtraining can emerge, such as persistent soreness, irritability, and plateaued progress.

Inflammation and Joint Impact

Inflammation often affects joints, tendons, and connective tissue, making them more sensitive to impact. High-intensity workouts like running or plyometrics place repeated stress on these areas, potentially aggravating pain and slowing healing. Even strength training, while beneficial in moderation, can backfire if form is compromised or recovery between sessions is insufficient. When tissues are inflamed, microtears take longer to repair, increasing the risk of injury and prolonging discomfort.

Lower-impact movement can still provide cardiovascular and muscular benefits without adding unnecessary strain. Activities like walking, swimming, cycling at an easy pace, or gentle yoga improve circulation and mobility while supporting the lymphatic system in clearing inflammatory byproducts. These forms of exercise are particularly helpful during the early phases of a healing protocol, when the body needs calm signals rather than additional challenges.

Recognizing when exercise is becoming counterproductive starts with listening to the body's feedback. Persistent fatigue, restless sleep, increased soreness, or difficulty recovering from workouts are signs that the nervous system is overwhelmed. Some people also notice increased cravings, mood swings, or unexplained weight fluctuations, all of which indicate stress hormones are staying elevated instead of returning to baseline after activity. When these patterns emerge, scaling back intensity or volume is often more beneficial than pushing harder.

An inflamed body often needs movement that supports circulation and mobility without creating additional stress. Low to moderate activities like walking outdoors, gentle yoga, tai chi, or swimming allow the body to remain active while prioritizing recovery. These movements help regulate blood sugar, improve lymphatic flow, and calm the nervous system, which are essential for lowering inflammation. Over time, as energy stabilizes and signs of chronic stress diminish, more challenging forms of exercise can be gradually reintroduced.

Supporting exercise with proper recovery strategies is equally important. Adequate sleep, nutrient-dense meals, and hydration provide the resources muscles and connective tissues need to repair. Incorporating stretching, breathwork, or relaxation techniques after workouts helps shift the body from fight-or-flight to rest-and-digest mode. This intentional transition reduces lingering cortisol and allows repair processes to unfold more efficiently.

Mindset also plays a role. Many people equate health with pushing harder — more miles, more weight, more sweat — and feel guilty when advised to slow down. Understanding that healing is cyclical, with periods of intensity followed by restoration, reframes recovery as a productive part of progress rather than a setback. Inflammation signals that the body is asking for gentler inputs; respecting this message often leads to faster and more sustainable improvements.

Over time, as inflammation resolves, the body responds differently to exercise. Workouts that once left you drained begin to feel energizing, and progress becomes steady rather than erratic. Building strength and cardiovascular fitness on a foundation of reduced inflammation not only improves performance but also protects against future injuries and energy crashes. Movement returns to its intended role — a tool for vitality and resilience rather than a source of additional stress.

When exercise is aligned with the body's current state, it becomes medicine rather than a burden. Healing accelerates, energy rises, and physical activity once again supports rather than sabotages well-being. This approach turns movement into a long-term ally, ensuring that it remains sustainable through every phase of life and health.

Gentle, Restorative Movement: Walking, Mobility, Strength Basics

Movement does not need to be extreme to be transformative. In fact, for a body recovering from chronic stress or inflammation, gentle and consistent activity often produces better results than high-intensity workouts. Walking, basic mobility drills, and foundational strength work provide circulation, stability, and resilience without overwhelming the nervous system. This approach builds a base of physical capacity that supports healing and prepares the body for more demanding activity later, should it be desired.

The Power of Walking

Walking is one of the most underestimated tools for healing. It improves cardiovascular health, supports lymphatic drainage, and enhances blood flow to muscles and joints, all while keeping stress hormones low. Unlike intense exercise, walking does not deplete energy stores or trigger strong hunger signals, making it sustainable even on days when fatigue is present.

Walking outdoors adds additional benefits. Sunlight exposure helps regulate circadian rhythms, improving sleep quality and mood. Contact with nature reduces stress responses in the brain and lowers blood pressure. Even short walks — ten to fifteen minutes after meals or during breaks — help stabilize blood sugar and reduce post-meal inflammation. Over time, daily walking becomes a cornerstone habit that reinforces nearly every aspect of recovery.

Mobility for Joint Health

Mobility exercises target the health of joints and connective tissue, which often suffer when the body has been under prolonged stress. Gentle range-of-motion drills — such as controlled shoulder circles, hip openers, and spinal rotations — keep joints lubricated and prevent stiffness from developing into pain or injury. These movements also improve body awareness, helping you notice areas of tension or imbalance that may need attention.

Incorporating mobility work into daily life does not require long sessions. A few minutes in the morning or evening, or short breaks throughout the day, are enough to maintain flexibility and prevent discomfort. Over time, mobility practice prepares the body for strength training by ensuring joints move freely and muscles can activate properly without compensation or strain.

Strength Basics Without Overload

Strength training supports bone density, metabolic health, and hormonal balance, but in an inflamed body, the approach must be measured. The goal at this stage is not maximal lifting or exhaustive workouts but reintroducing basic patterns that build stability: squats, hinges, pushes, pulls, and carries. These movements can be performed with body weight or light resistance to start, emphasizing proper form and controlled tempo over intensity.

Integrating walking, mobility, and basic strength work into a routine does not require hours a day or complex programming. Consistency and gradual progression are the keys to success. Starting with short, manageable sessions — perhaps a 15-minute walk, five minutes of mobility drills, and two to three simple strength exercises — allows the body to adapt without becoming overwhelmed. As endurance and comfort grow, these sessions can lengthen or increase in intensity, always prioritizing how the body feels and recovers.

Recovery between sessions is critical. Listening to signs of fatigue or soreness helps prevent overtraining, which can reignite inflammation and stall progress. Adequate sleep, hydration, and nutrition provide the foundation for repair, while gentle stretching or breathwork on rest days promotes circulation and nervous system calm. Rest does not mean inactivity but intentional self-care that supports movement habits.

The mental aspect of movement should not be underestimated. Approaching exercise with curiosity and compassion transforms it from a chore into an opportunity for connection with the body. Noticing improvements in mobility, strength, or endurance provides motivation, while gentle self-encouragement during setbacks builds resilience. This mindset shift encourages sustainable habits that become part of a lifestyle rather than a temporary fix.

For those new to movement or recovering from significant health challenges, working with a qualified professional — such as a physical therapist, trainer, or movement coach — can provide personalized guidance. These experts help ensure exercises are performed safely, tailor progressions appropriately, and address any underlying movement limitations or imbalances. Professional support accelerates recovery and builds confidence in the body's abilities.

Ultimately, gentle and restorative movement creates a positive feedback loop. Improved mobility and strength reduce pain and stiffness, making daily tasks easier and more enjoyable. Increased circulation and oxygenation support healing at the cellular level. Enhanced body awareness fosters better posture and movement patterns, which protect against injury and chronic pain. These benefits reinforce each other, making movement an accessible, effective, and empowering tool for health.

By prioritizing gentle movement during healing, you honor the body's current state while building capacity for greater vitality. This approach not only supports the reset protocol but lays the groundwork for lifelong physical well-being. Movement becomes medicine — a source of strength, calm, and resilience that complements every other aspect of your health journey.

Building a Sustainable Movement Plan for Energy and Longevity

Creating a movement plan that supports energy and longevity requires a shift in perspective. Exercise is not just about burning calories or building muscle; it is about nourishing the body's capacity to function well over decades. This means designing routines that are enjoyable, adaptable, and balanced — prioritizing consistent engagement rather than intensity or perfection. A sustainable plan fosters resilience, reduces inflammation, and enhances quality of life without creating additional stress.

Understanding Your Starting Point

Every body is unique, and sustainable movement begins with an honest assessment of your current state. This includes energy levels, mobility, any existing injuries or limitations, and how you feel during and after different types of activity. For some, this might mean starting with daily walks and gentle stretching; for others, it could include more structured strength training or cardiovascular work. Recognizing where you are sets realistic expectations and prevents overambition that can lead to burnout.

Balancing Intensity and Recovery

Sustainability depends on balancing activity with rest. Movement should challenge the body enough to stimulate adaptation but not so much that it triggers excessive fatigue or inflammation. Recovery practices like quality sleep, hydration, and nutrition are as essential as the workouts themselves. The goal is to create a rhythm of stress and restoration that the body can thrive within — this balance enhances mitochondrial function, hormonal regulation, and immune resilience, all vital for longevity.

Incorporating Variety

Variety keeps movement engaging and addresses multiple facets of health. Combining cardiovascular exercise, strength training, mobility work, and balance challenges different systems, preventing overuse injuries and promoting holistic fitness. Mixing activities also maintains motivation, reducing the risk of boredom or mental fatigue. For example, alternating walking, swimming, yoga, and resistance exercises throughout the week offers a well-rounded approach that supports energy and long-term health.

Designing a weekly framework begins with identifying non-negotiable habits rather than packing in as many workouts as possible. Even two or three sessions that combine gentle strength training and cardiovascular work can be enough at first, especially if supported by daily walking or light mobility exercises. Over time, volume and intensity can increase naturally as energy improves and inflammation subsides. The emphasis is on progression that feels supportive rather than punishing.

Consistency matters more than perfection. Missing a session occasionally does not derail progress; what matters is returning to the routine without guilt and maintaining overall patterns over months and years. This mindset removes the all-or-nothing pressure that leads many people to quit when life becomes busy. Viewing movement as part of daily living — walking to do errands, stretching between tasks, using stairs instead of elevators — turns exercise into a lifestyle rather than an isolated chore.

Sustainable plans also adapt to changing circumstances. Stressful weeks may require lighter sessions or more mobility work, while periods of higher energy allow for increased intensity or exploring new activities. Listening to the body and adjusting accordingly prevents burnout and supports long-term adherence. This flexibility is especially important for those recovering from chronic inflammation, where energy levels can fluctuate as healing progresses.

Environmental and social factors enhance sustainability as well. Training outdoors when possible improves mood and vitamin D levels, while exercising with a friend or group adds accountability and enjoyment.

Creating a designated space at home for bodyweight training or yoga makes movement more accessible and reduces friction in maintaining consistency.

Tracking progress can provide motivation but should focus on functional improvements rather than aesthetics. Increased energy, reduced stiffness, better sleep, and improved mood are valuable indicators of success that often appear before visible physical changes. Celebrating these milestones reinforces positive behavior and helps shift the goal from appearance to vitality and longevity.

Ultimately, a sustainable movement plan blends structure with intuition. It builds capacity gradually, respects recovery, and evolves with your life rather than competing with it. When aligned with the body's needs, movement becomes a source of stability and energy, laying a foundation for resilience well into the future. This approach transforms exercise from a short-term fix into a lifelong practice that supports healing, vitality, and a deep sense of well-being.

Part IV. Living the Protocol for Life

Healing is not just about completing a reset or following a structured program for a few weeks. The real transformation happens when the principles you have practiced become part of daily living. This final part of the book is about integration — carrying forward what you have learned so that health is no longer a struggle, but a natural outcome of the way you live.

By now, you understand how inflammation, hormones, gut health, and the nervous system interact. You have seen how removing triggers, nourishing the body, and adopting restorative habits can create profound shifts in energy and resilience. The next step is to sustain these gains without falling into extremes. This means adapting the protocol to the realities of everyday life — busy schedules, travel, celebrations, and inevitable periods of stress — while maintaining the core habits that support balance.

Living the protocol for life is not about rigid rules or constant vigilance. It is about knowing your body well enough to recognize what helps and what harms, and having the tools to adjust when life changes. Some weeks may look near perfect, while others may be more flexible. Both are acceptable, because health is built on consistency over time, not momentary perfection.

This part will guide you through strategies to maintain vitality long term: how to prevent relapse into old patterns, how to handle setbacks with perspective, and how to evolve your habits as your goals and life circumstances shift. It will help you transition from short-term healing to lifelong resilience, where the reset becomes a way of being rather than a program you complete.

When these principles are fully integrated, you no longer have to think of health as something separate from life. It becomes part of how you eat, move, rest, and connect — a foundation that allows you to pursue everything else with clarity and energy. This is the point where healing turns into thriving, and where the benefits of your effort compound for years to come.

Chapter 10: Detoxing Your Environment

The Toxins Hiding in Your Home (and How to Remove Them)

Many people associate toxins with industrial sites or pollution outside their door, yet some of the most significant exposures occur inside the home. Modern living has introduced thousands of synthetic chemicals into everyday products — cleaning supplies, cookware, furniture, and even the air we breathe indoors. These compounds are often invisible and odorless, yet they can contribute to low-level inflammation, disrupt hormones, and burden detox systems over time. Understanding where they hide is the first step toward reducing exposure and creating a home that supports healing rather than undermines it.

Indoor Air Quality and Volatile Compounds

Indoor air often contains more pollutants than outdoor air, largely because of off-gassing from building materials, furniture, and household products. Volatile organic compounds (VOCs) are chemicals released from items like paint, carpets, adhesives, and cleaning agents. Prolonged exposure has been linked to headaches, respiratory irritation, and hormone disruption. Poor ventilation compounds the problem, trapping these substances inside.

Improving air quality does not require expensive purifiers, although those can help. Simple actions like opening windows regularly, using exhaust fans, and incorporating houseplants known for filtering air can make a noticeable difference. Choosing low-VOC paints and finishes during renovations and allowing new furniture to off-gas outdoors or in well-ventilated areas before use further reduces exposure.

Plastics in the Kitchen

The kitchen is another major source of hidden toxins, especially through plastics used for food storage and cooking. Compounds like BPA and phthalates can leach into food and beverages, particularly when plastics are heated or scratched. These chemicals mimic hormones in the body, potentially contributing to reproductive issues and metabolic imbalances.

Switching to glass, stainless steel, or high-quality silicone for storage and cookware is a practical step. Avoid microwaving food in plastic containers or using single-use plastic water bottles when possible. Even small swaps — like choosing wooden cutting boards instead of plastic or stainless-steel water bottles over disposable ones — significantly lower daily exposure.

Cleaning Products and Synthetic Fragrances

Household cleaners and air fresheners are marketed as creating a fresh, safe home, yet many contain harsh solvents, synthetic fragrances, and endocrine-disrupting chemicals. These substances are inhaled during use and linger on surfaces long after. Repeated exposure, even at low levels, adds up over time, particularly in households with children or pets.

Natural alternatives like vinegar, baking soda, and unscented castile soap provide effective cleaning without harmful residues. For those who prefer fragrance, essential oils can replace synthetic scents without introducing toxic compounds. Reading ingredient labels and choosing products labeled fragrance-free or non-toxic can dramatically reduce chemical load without sacrificing cleanliness.

Furniture and household textiles can be another overlooked source of toxins. Flame retardants and stain-resistant chemicals, commonly used in couches, mattresses, and rugs, release particles into household dust that are inhaled or ingested over time. These compounds have been associated with hormonal disruption and developmental concerns, particularly in children. Choosing natural materials like untreated cotton, wool, or solid wood when replacing items reduces future exposure. For existing furniture, frequent vacuuming with a HEPA filter and wet dusting surfaces can limit the buildup of contaminated dust in living spaces.

Personal care products contribute to cumulative exposure as well. Lotions, shampoos, and cosmetics often contain parabens, phthalates, and synthetic fragrances that absorb through the skin and enter the bloodstream. Unlike food, these products bypass digestion and detox pathways, meaning even small daily amounts can add up. Transitioning to simpler formulas with short ingredient lists and avoiding products that list "fragrance" without specifying its source is a practical approach. Over time, these swaps support hormone balance and reduce unnecessary chemical load without requiring a complete overhaul of routines.

Household dust itself often holds a mix of these compounds — flame retardants, microplastics, pesticide residues — because they accumulate in fabrics and settle over time. Regular cleaning strategies can mitigate this hidden risk. Using a vacuum with a HEPA filter, dusting with a damp cloth instead of a dry one, and frequently washing bedding and curtains help keep these particles from recirculating. These small habits create a noticeably cleaner and safer environment without requiring significant expense or specialized products.

Water quality is another factor often overlooked in home toxin exposure. Tap water can carry trace amounts of heavy metals, chlorine byproducts, and pesticide residues depending on local sources and infrastructure. While municipal water is generally safe from acute harm, chronic exposure to low levels of contaminants may contribute to inflammation over time. Installing a quality water filter suited to your local water report — whether a simple carbon filter or a more advanced reverse osmosis system — reduces this burden significantly and supports the body's detox pathways.

Addressing toxins in the home is not about striving for perfection or creating fear around everyday items. It is about making gradual, strategic changes that lower the overall load on the body's detox systems. Each swap, from storing leftovers in glass containers to choosing fragrance-free cleaners, contributes to an environment that supports healing rather than undermines it. Over months, these changes compound, creating a home that feels lighter, cleaner, and more aligned with your health goals. By approaching toxin reduction as an ongoing process rather than a single overhaul, it becomes sustainable. Every adjustment improves resilience and helps the body focus on repair rather than constant defense. This shift allows the benefits of other protocol steps — nourishing foods, restorative movement, and stress regulation — to work more effectively, setting the stage for long-term vitality and well-being.

Water, Air, and Household Products That Support Healing

Healing is not only about removing harmful exposures but also about actively creating an environment that nurtures the body. The water you drink, the air you breathe, and the products you use every day can either enhance the healing process or subtly work against it. By choosing supportive alternatives, you give your body fewer obstacles to manage and more space to repair, restore, and thrive.

Water Quality and Hydration

Water is central to every cellular function, from digestion to detoxification. Yet tap water in many areas contains chlorine, fluoride, trace pesticides, or even heavy metals from aging infrastructure. While these levels are typically regulated for safety, long-term exposure can still tax the body's detox systems, particularly if other environmental stresses are present.

Filtering water does not need to be complicated or expensive. A basic carbon filter can remove chlorine and improve taste, while more advanced systems like reverse osmosis or multi-stage filters can reduce a broader range of contaminants. The best choice depends on your local water report, which outlines the specific impurities in your supply. Knowing what is in your water allows you to select the most efficient solution without unnecessary cost or complexity.

Beyond filtration, how water is stored also matters. Using stainless steel or glass containers avoids the leaching of chemicals from plastic bottles, especially when exposed to heat or sunlight. These simple shifts provide cleaner hydration and reduce the body's daily chemical burden without requiring dramatic lifestyle changes.

Breathing Cleaner Indoor Air

Indoor air quality often receives less attention than food or water, yet we inhale thousands of liters of air daily. Dust, pet dander, mold spores, and volatile organic compounds from furniture or cleaning products accumulate indoors, particularly in poorly ventilated spaces. Over time, these exposures can contribute to respiratory irritation, headaches, or low-grade inflammation.

Improving indoor air does not necessarily require sophisticated equipment. Regularly opening windows to circulate fresh air, vacuuming with HEPA filters, and avoiding synthetic air fresheners are simple habits with measurable impact. Houseplants like spider plants or peace lilies can also contribute by absorbing certain airborne compounds, although they are supplemental rather than a primary solution. For those in urban areas or with allergies, an air purifier with a high-efficiency filter can further reduce particulate matter and allergens, creating a calmer environment for the respiratory and immune systems.

Household products often determine whether the home supports healing or contributes to a steady stream of low-level toxins. Cleaning supplies are one of the most common culprits, as many conventional formulas contain harsh solvents, bleach, or synthetic fragrances that linger in the air and on surfaces. These chemicals may irritate the respiratory system or disrupt hormones when used regularly. Choosing simpler alternatives, like unscented castile soap, vinegar, or baking soda, reduces this exposure while still maintaining cleanliness. For targeted disinfecting, options such as diluted hydrogen peroxide provide effectiveness without unnecessary additives.

Personal care products deserve equal attention. Lotions, shampoos, deodorants, and cosmetics are absorbed through the skin and can introduce compounds like parabens, phthalates, and synthetic musks. Over time, these add to the body's chemical load. Transitioning to products with transparent ingredient lists, prioritizing unscented or naturally scented options, and simplifying routines where possible can reduce cumulative exposure. It is not about replacing everything at once but about gradually shifting toward choices that align with the body's natural healing processes.

Even seemingly minor items, such as candles or laundry detergents, can affect indoor air quality and skin health. Many fragranced candles release soot and chemicals as they burn, while detergents often leave residues that can irritate sensitive skin. Opting for beeswax or soy candles without added fragrance and detergents free of dyes or perfumes creates a calmer, cleaner home environment. These small adjustments contribute to a larger shift in how the body experiences its surroundings.

Creating a healing space also involves mindful purchasing decisions for future items. Furniture, bedding, and cookware can be selected with an eye toward natural materials and durability rather than convenience or lowest cost. Solid wood furniture, organic cotton linens, and stainless-steel cookware are often safer long-term investments than particleboard, synthetic fabrics, or nonstick coatings that may degrade over time and release harmful compounds.

The cumulative effect of these changes is significant. While each adjustment may seem small on its own, together they lower the body's daily burden and free energy for repair and recovery. This supportive environment allows the other elements of the protocol — nutrition, movement, stress management — to work more effectively. Over time, the home becomes not just a place to live but an active partner in maintaining vitality and resilience.

Prioritizing cleaner water, fresher air, and safer household products is less about perfection than about alignment. It is about giving your body an environment where its natural healing mechanisms can operate without interference. With each intentional choice, you create a space that nourishes rather than drains, setting the stage for long-term health and a life that feels lighter, calmer, and more sustainable.

Creating a Low-Toxin Lifestyle Without Overwhelm or Perfectionism

Lowering daily exposure to toxins is one of the most impactful ways to reduce chronic inflammation and support healing, but it is also where many people become discouraged. The modern world is full of chemicals — in food packaging, personal care, cleaning products, furniture — and attempting to eliminate every single one can quickly lead to frustration or burnout. The goal is not to live in a bubble or chase perfection. It is to make consistent, sustainable changes that reduce the body's overall burden without creating stress or fear in the process.

Shifting the Mindset Around Toxins

The first step in building a low-toxin lifestyle is approaching the topic with perspective rather than panic. It is true that environmental toxins can accumulate and influence health, but the body also has remarkable detoxification systems designed to handle reasonable exposure. Supporting these systems through better choices enhances resilience rather than aiming for an impossible standard of zero exposure. This mindset shift reframes the process as empowering rather than restrictive, turning it into a positive act of self-care rather than a constant battle.

Start with the Big Wins

Not all changes have equal impact. Certain exposures, like drinking water quality or heavily fragranced cleaning products, contribute more significantly to the daily toxic load than others. Focusing on these higher-impact areas first creates noticeable benefits without requiring a total overhaul of your life. Swapping plastic food containers for glass, replacing conventional household cleaners with simpler options, or installing a basic water filter are examples of small, high-leverage steps that set the foundation for gradual improvement.

Layering Changes Over Time

Attempting to replace every product in your home at once is overwhelming and rarely sustainable. A layered approach — addressing one area at a time — prevents decision fatigue and allows you to evaluate each change before moving on to the next. For example, start with kitchen items, then shift to personal care, followed by cleaning supplies. Each step builds confidence and momentum, turning the transition into a natural evolution rather than a rigid overhaul.

Evaluating products becomes easier when you focus on simplicity rather than marketing claims. A shorter ingredient list is often a sign of fewer unnecessary additives, and items without synthetic fragrances or dyes generally reduce exposure to common irritants. Trusted third-party certifications, like organic or EWG-verified labels, can provide additional reassurance, but they are not always necessary for making better choices. Reading labels gradually builds familiarity, turning what once felt confusing into a habit that requires little extra thought over time.

Managing costs is another concern that can create stress if not addressed directly. Healthier options sometimes appear more expensive at first glance, but many swaps save money long term. Using vinegar and baking soda for cleaning, for example, is significantly cheaper than buying multiple specialized products. Choosing reusable containers instead of disposable ones reduces waste and recurring costs. Focusing on gradual replacement rather than immediate overhaul prevents financial strain and helps prioritize changes that deliver the greatest benefits for the investment.

Avoiding perfectionism is key to sustaining a low-toxin lifestyle. It is unrealistic to expect a completely chemical-free home, and occasional exposures will not undo your progress. Instead, measure success by overall improvement rather than absolutes. If ninety percent of your daily environment supports healing, the body can easily manage the small exposures that remain. This flexible approach prevents feelings of failure and allows you to adapt as life circumstances change, such as during travel, busy work periods, or family events.

Staying consistent over the long term involves returning to why these changes matter. Noticing tangible benefits — clearer energy, fewer headaches, calmer digestion — reinforces motivation. Over time, these shifts become less about what you are avoiding and more about how good it feels to live in alignment with your health goals. The process stops feeling like a project and starts feeling like your normal way of life. A low-toxin lifestyle is ultimately about balance. It creates a supportive environment without demanding rigid control, allowing space for enjoyment and flexibility. As new habits solidify, they free mental energy for other priorities, from relationships to personal growth. The focus moves from fear of harm toward trust in your body's ability to thrive when given the right conditions. This mindset transforms toxin reduction from an overwhelming task into a sustainable framework that quietly supports vitality every day.

Chapter 11: Living the Protocol for Life

Building a Long-Term System of Self-Healing

Healing is not a one-time event but an ongoing process. The goal is not only to recover from inflammation, fatigue, or imbalance but to create a personal framework that keeps you resilient in the face of life's inevitable stressors. A self-healing system combines awareness, daily habits, and adaptability, allowing you to respond quickly to early warning signs rather than waiting for small issues to become major problems.

Cultivating Awareness

The foundation of self-healing is knowing your body well enough to recognize subtle shifts before they escalate. This means paying attention to energy levels, digestion, mood, and sleep quality. These signals are feedback loops — early indicators of whether your lifestyle choices are supporting or straining your system. By regularly tuning in rather than ignoring discomfort, you can make small course corrections instead of resorting to dramatic interventions later.

Awareness also includes understanding personal triggers. For some, stress might show up first as poor sleep or sugar cravings; for others, it may appear as joint stiffness or brain fog. Identifying these patterns helps you predict and prevent flare-ups, empowering you to act early rather than feeling blindsided when symptoms intensify.

Designing Core Daily Habits

A sustainable self-healing system rests on simple daily actions that create stability. Consistent meal timing, hydration, restorative movement, and quality sleep provide the body with predictable rhythms that reduce stress and optimize recovery. These habits do not need to be complicated; in fact, simplicity often makes them more effective and easier to maintain.

Nutrition centered around whole foods, paired with moderate physical activity like walking or gentle strength training, sets a strong baseline. Combined with practices that calm the nervous system — deep breathing, short breaks outdoors, or mindful transitions between work and rest — these habits build a body that is more resistant to inflammation and better equipped to handle challenges.

Reinforcing habits over time requires building them into a structure that feels natural rather than forced. This might involve creating morning or evening routines that anchor the day. A few minutes of movement upon waking, preparing nourishing meals in advance, or setting reminders for hydration can transform small actions into automatic behaviors. By reducing decision fatigue, these structures free up mental energy for more important choices while ensuring your core practices remain consistent.

Periodic reflection is equally important. Checking in weekly or monthly helps you notice patterns that may otherwise go unseen. Journaling or simply observing changes in energy, mood, and physical comfort provides feedback on whether your habits are working or need adjustment. These check-ins prevent autopilot living and encourage curiosity about what your body is communicating at different phases of life.

Flexibility is what allows this system to last. Life will inevitably bring stress, travel, and unexpected demands. A rigid plan often collapses under pressure, while a flexible one adapts without losing its foundation. Instead of abandoning healthy habits during busy periods, you can scale them back — shorter walks, simpler meals, earlier bedtimes — maintaining continuity even when perfection is not possible. This mindset transforms challenges into opportunities to refine and deepen your self-healing approach.

Periodic resets can also play a role. These are not extreme detoxes or quick fixes, but intentional periods of recalibration when you notice drift in your habits or rising stress signals. A reset might mean dedicating a week to focus on sleep hygiene, simplifying meals, or spending more time outdoors. By pausing and realigning before imbalances worsen, you avoid cycles of depletion and recovery and stay closer to balance year-round.

Over time, this framework evolves with you. What worked in one season of life may need adjustment in another, and that is part of the process. The key is trusting your body's feedback and remaining open to refining your practices rather than clinging to rigid rules. This ongoing dialogue between awareness and action creates resilience — a dynamic balance that supports not only physical health but also mental clarity and emotional stability.

Ultimately, building a long-term system of self-healing is about creating conditions where health is maintained without constant struggle. It is about trusting that small, consistent actions accumulate and that responding early to the body's signals prevents crises before they arise. This foundation supports not just recovery from chronic inflammation but a way of living that prioritizes vitality, balance, and the freedom to engage fully with life's demands and opportunities.

How to Listen to Your Body and Adjust Over Time

One of the most powerful skills for long-term health is learning to read your body's signals and respond before small imbalances turn into bigger problems. Many people are taught to override discomfort — push through fatigue, ignore cravings, dismiss pain — until symptoms become severe enough to demand medical intervention. Rebuilding trust with your body involves unlearning this habit and replacing it with attentive awareness, curiosity, and timely adjustments.

Recognizing the Language of the Body

Your body communicates constantly through sensations and subtle changes. Energy levels, digestion, sleep quality, skin clarity, and even mood shifts all reflect the state of your internal systems. When inflammation rises, you might notice increased stiffness, bloating, or irritability. When hormones are imbalanced, fatigue, cravings, or disrupted sleep can appear. Rather than labeling these as random or inconvenient, they can be treated as valuable feedback.

Recognizing patterns is key. A single poor night's sleep may not mean much, but consistent restlessness can point toward stress or dietary triggers. Occasional digestive discomfort might be normal, but recurring symptoms signal the need for closer attention. By tracking how lifestyle factors — food choices, movement, stress, environment — affect these patterns, you begin to connect cause and effect more clearly.

The Role of Curiosity Rather Than Judgment

Listening to your body is less about strict analysis and more about cultivating curiosity. Instead of judging yourself for feeling tired or bloated, you approach it as a clue. What changed recently? Was it stress, hydration, sleep, or something in your diet? This mindset removes shame and turns self-care into an experiment, where you learn and adjust rather than criticize. Over time, this curiosity develops into a quiet confidence: you trust your ability to understand and respond to what your body needs.

Daily Check-Ins and Subtle Adjustments

Small daily check-ins build this awareness into routine. Asking yourself simple questions — How is my energy? Do I feel clear-headed or foggy? Am I hungry, or just bored? — keeps you connected to your internal cues. From there, adjustments can be small and targeted: drinking more water if thirst is consistent, adding rest if soreness lingers, or scaling back caffeine if sleep is disrupted. These course corrections prevent small imbalances from snowballing and keep you aligned with your body's needs.

As life evolves, so do the signals your body sends. Stress at work, changes in sleep schedules, travel, or new dietary patterns can all alter how your body responds. Developing a long-term relationship with these signals allows you to adapt without anxiety. Instead of fearing setbacks, you learn to treat them as information. When energy dips or digestion falters, you can pause, identify contributing factors, and make small corrections before deeper issues emerge.

Adapting habits seasonally is especially valuable. Colder months may require more grounding foods, extra hydration, or gentle movement to maintain circulation, while warmer months might invite lighter meals and outdoor activity. These shifts align with natural rhythms and reduce strain on your body. Paying attention to how your energy and mood change across these cycles helps refine your approach without the need for strict rules or constant monitoring.

Feedback loops create resilience over time. Each time you adjust based on your body's cues and see improvement, you strengthen the connection between awareness and trust. You begin to rely less on external advice and more on your own observations. This internal guidance becomes the backbone of sustainable health — flexible, personal, and responsive rather than rigid or prescriptive.

Avoiding hyper-vigilance is equally important. Being tuned in to your body should not mean obsessing over every small sensation or fearing occasional discomfort. Minor fluctuations are part of life and do not always signal a problem. The key is to discern patterns and respond thoughtfully rather than react impulsively. This balanced approach allows you to remain present and engaged in life without being consumed by self-monitoring.

Over months and years, this practice transforms your relationship with health. Instead of chasing quick fixes or rigid programs, you create a lifestyle that adapts naturally to your needs. You know when to push and when to rest, when to simplify and when to expand. This dynamic awareness not only prevents relapse into old habits but fosters confidence that you can handle whatever challenges arise. Listening to your body in this way turns healing from a temporary goal into a lifelong skill — one that evolves alongside you and supports every stage of your life.

From Survival to Thriving: Redefining What "Healthy" Means

For many people, the concept of health is tied to absence of disease — a body free of obvious symptoms or lab results that fall within normal ranges. But this definition is limited. It frames health as something static, achieved once and maintained only by avoiding illness. In reality, true health is dynamic. It is not just surviving but thriving — having the energy, clarity, and resilience to fully engage with life rather than simply endure it.

Moving Beyond Symptom Management

Modern healthcare often focuses on managing symptoms rather than addressing root causes. Fatigue is treated with stimulants, pain with anti-inflammatories, sleep problems with sedatives. While these interventions can provide relief, they rarely create lasting vitality. Thriving requires identifying why symptoms arise in the first place — whether from stress, inflammation, nutrient depletion, or environmental factors — and working to restore balance at the source.

This shift from survival to thriving transforms how you approach daily decisions. Instead of asking "How can I stop feeling bad?" you begin to ask "What will help me feel my best?" This subtle reframe encourages proactive choices — nourishing meals, restorative movement, supportive environments — that create upward momentum rather than temporary relief.

The Role of Energy and Clarity

Energy is one of the clearest indicators of whether you are thriving or merely getting by. Thriving energy feels steady and reliable, supporting focus and motivation without constant crashes or dependence on stimulants. Clarity, both mental and emotional, is equally vital. A thriving state allows you to respond to challenges with calm rather than reactivity, and to enjoy life's moments rather than simply endure them.

Achieving this state is not about perfection. It is about stacking habits and environments that consistently support your body's needs so that vitality becomes the default rather than the exception. This creates a sense of ease — health no longer feels like a project but rather the natural outcome of how you live day to day.

Thriving begins with building stability in the fundamentals — food, rest, movement, emotional balance — but it does not end there. Once the body's systems are supported and inflammation is lowered, there is space to ask deeper questions. What brings meaning? What fuels creativity? What relationships or environments enhance a sense of belonging? These layers of fulfillment are part of health too, even though they are rarely measured in lab tests or addressed in standard treatment plans.

Thriving health also changes how you handle challenges. Stressors and setbacks will still arise, but the difference lies in recovery. A thriving body bounces back faster, using stress as a temporary signal rather than a permanent drain. Mental resilience improves as well; self-care becomes instinctive rather than forced. Instead of fearing that one poor meal, late night, or busy week will undo progress, you trust your system to recalibrate because you have built a strong foundation.

This redefinition of health shifts motivation from fear to possibility. You are no longer making choices solely to avoid illness; you are choosing what allows you to live fully. The focus moves from restriction to abundance — nourishing foods because they help you feel vibrant, daily movement because it clears your mind and keeps you strong, rest because it sharpens your focus and helps you show up better in life.

Over time, this mindset fosters a profound sense of freedom. You no longer chase quick fixes or rigid plans because your daily life already supports how you want to feel. Health is no longer separate from living but woven into every part of it — how you work, connect, and care for yourself. That shift marks the difference between surviving and thriving. It turns wellness into a dynamic, lifelong practice that evolves with you and enriches every moment of your experience.

Chapter 12: Beyond the Reset.
Advanced Strategies for Lifelong Healing

The Mindset That Keeps You Healing

The shift from temporary change to lasting transformation begins in the mind. Most people approach health protocols with short-term intensity — an initial surge of motivation fueled by discomfort or fear — only to burn out when results slow or life disrupts routines. Long-term healing demands a different mindset: one grounded in patience, flexibility, and trust in the body's process. This mental shift turns the protocol from something you do into something you live.

From Urgency to Stewardship

At the start of any healing journey, urgency is common. Symptoms feel unbearable, and the desire for relief can drive strict adherence to new routines. While urgency can spark action, it cannot sustain it. Healing is rarely linear; there are plateaus, setbacks, and subtle improvements that may not feel dramatic day to day. A sustainable mindset replaces urgency with stewardship — the understanding that you are caring for your body over the long haul, like tending a garden rather than fighting a fire.
Stewardship changes how you evaluate progress. Instead of obsessing over quick fixes, you begin to notice gradual patterns: better energy in the mornings, fewer cravings, improved recovery from stress. These are quiet markers of healing, easy to miss if you are looking for instant transformation. Cultivating patience allows you to value these signs and stay committed even when the changes feel subtle.

Redefining Success

A mindset that sustains healing redefines what success looks like. It is no longer measured solely by the absence of symptoms but by an increasing sense of resilience and adaptability. Success is having the capacity to handle a stressful week without spiraling into exhaustion, or enjoying a meal with friends without anxiety about perfect food choices. It is about reclaiming trust in your body's ability to rebound rather than living in fear of setbacks.

This redefinition frees you from perfectionism. Perfection implies failure at the first deviation, which often leads to abandoning the protocol entirely. Resilience means acknowledging fluctuations and continuing forward regardless. Progress is measured in seasons, not days. When you expect healing to evolve over time, patience and consistency become more natural, and the pressure of unrealistic timelines dissolves.

Identity and Self-Compassion

True change sticks when it becomes part of who you are, not just something you do. If health remains an external goal — a task on your to-do list — it is fragile. When it becomes part of your identity — "I am someone who supports my body" — it is durable. This shift happens gradually as small habits reinforce a new self-image: choosing nourishing meals, prioritizing rest, moving daily. Each choice affirms the identity of someone who values and protects their well-being.

Self-compassion is essential in this process. Healing can bring frustration, especially when old patterns resurface. Without compassion, setbacks trigger shame and self-criticism, which erode motivation. With compassion, setbacks become opportunities to learn and adjust. The difference is subtle but powerful: shame pushes you away from awareness, while compassion invites you to stay present and curious. Over time, this soft persistence creates more stability than harsh self-discipline ever could.

Practical strategies help make this mindset tangible rather than abstract. One of the most effective is focusing on small wins. Instead of waiting for dramatic breakthroughs, you look for incremental improvements — sleeping through the night more often, clearer concentration in the mornings, less tension after stressful days. Acknowledging these shifts reinforces motivation and reminds you that healing is cumulative.

Rituals also anchor the mindset. Simple daily practices like checking in with your energy levels, preparing a nourishing meal, or spending time outdoors create rhythm and predictability. These rituals act as quiet affirmations of your commitment and reduce decision fatigue. Over time, they become automatic, freeing mental space for deeper healing rather than constant self-monitoring.

Learning to navigate setbacks is another crucial element. Healing is rarely a straight line; life events, stress, or unavoidable exposures will create fluctuations. The difference between people who maintain progress and those who abandon it often lies in how they interpret these moments. Instead of viewing a setback as failure, you can see it as feedback. What triggered the shift? What adjustment is needed? This approach transforms obstacles into information rather than excuses to quit.

Support structures enhance resilience as well. Sharing your journey with someone you trust, whether a friend, partner, or support group, can provide perspective when motivation wanes. Even a brief conversation can remind you of how far you've come and why the work matters. This external encouragement complements the internal mindset you are building, creating a balance between personal responsibility and communal support.

Over time, the mindset becomes less about managing symptoms and more about living in alignment with what nourishes you. The focus shifts from avoiding harm to cultivating strength and clarity. This is what makes healing sustainable — it stops feeling like a burden and begins to feel like freedom. The daily choices you make are no longer about restriction but about building a life that supports your energy, focus, and capacity to thrive.

When this shift takes root, the protocol becomes second nature. Habits no longer feel like chores because they align with who you are becoming. Challenges still arise, but they no longer derail you; they simply invite you to recalibrate and continue forward. This is the mindset that carries healing into every stage of life — adaptable, compassionate, and quietly powerful.

Tracking and Personalizing Your Healing Journey

Healing is rarely identical for two people. Even when following the same protocol, unique factors — genetics, environment, stress levels, and history — shape how the body responds. This is why tracking and personalizing your approach is vital. Without it, progress can feel vague or uncertain, leading to discouragement or unnecessary changes. With it, you gain clarity on what works, where adjustments are needed, and how far you've come.

Why Tracking Matters

Healing from chronic inflammation often involves subtle shifts before dramatic improvements. Energy stabilizes, sleep deepens, digestion improves — yet without tracking, these gains can be overlooked. Human memory tends to fixate on discomfort, so small wins are easily forgotten. A structured record creates perspective, transforming the process from guesswork to informed decision-making. It also prevents overcorrection; rather than abandoning a strategy too soon, you can see measurable trends that guide next steps.

Tracking also strengthens motivation. Seeing patterns emerge — fewer headaches, more restful mornings, steadier moods — reminds you that the work is paying off. Even when progress feels slow, the data shows forward movement, encouraging consistency through challenging phases of the protocol.

Simple Metrics That Matter

Effective tracking does not require complex spreadsheets or constant monitoring. The most valuable data points are often simple and directly tied to how you feel day to day. These include:

- **Energy levels:** A daily rating, such as 1 to 10, captures fluctuations and trends.
- **Sleep quality:** Recording how easily you fall asleep and how rested you feel on waking reveals connections between habits and rest.

- **Mood and mental clarity:** Notes on focus, irritability, or brain fog help identify triggers and improvements.
- **Digestive comfort:** Observing bloating, regularity, or food sensitivities highlights gut progress.

Optional additions, like body measurements, skin clarity, or physical stamina, can provide further insights without becoming overwhelming. The key is consistency rather than volume of data — choose a few markers you can realistically track over time.

Recognizing Patterns

Once basic data is collected, the next step is interpreting it. Look for recurring links between habits and outcomes. Does better hydration correlate with improved energy? Do late nights consistently precede inflammation flares? Does removing a certain food reduce brain fog? Identifying these patterns allows for informed adjustments rather than trial-and-error guesswork.

Personalization begins with identifying which elements of the protocol bring the most noticeable improvements. When you track energy, sleep, mood, and digestion consistently, certain patterns stand out. Maybe removing processed foods significantly reduces bloating but has less impact on sleep, or managing evening light exposure dramatically improves rest but requires consistency to maintain. These observations help prioritize what deserves the most attention and effort, creating a tailored plan that aligns with your body's specific responses rather than following generic advice.

Adjusting intensity is another part of personalization. Early in healing, more structure may be needed — deliberate meal planning, consistent sleep schedules, mindful tracking of stress. As the body stabilizes, some flexibility can be reintroduced without losing progress. For example, you may discover that occasional indulgences do not trigger symptoms once the foundation is strong, allowing you to live more freely while still honoring your body's limits.

Feedback loops make this process ongoing rather than static. Instead of rigidly following one version of the protocol forever, you periodically reassess: What symptoms have improved? Which habits feel sustainable? Where do flare-ups still occur? These questions prevent stagnation and ensure the approach evolves alongside changing needs, whether due to life transitions, stress, or seasonal shifts.

Some people benefit from integrating periodic check-ins with professionals. Functional or integrative practitioners can provide lab tests — hormone profiles, gut microbiome assessments, inflammation markers like CRP — that complement your self-observations. These tests are not essential for everyone but can offer deeper insight when progress plateaus or when personal tracking reveals persistent issues. Partnering with a professional can also provide reassurance that you are on the right path and prevent unnecessary experimentation.

Ultimately, the value of tracking and personalization is clarity. Instead of guessing why you feel better or worse, you develop a narrative supported by patterns and observations. This clarity reduces anxiety, builds confidence, and empowers you to adapt without fear. Over time, the practice becomes less about constant monitoring and more about intuition; you know what balance feels like and can sense when adjustments are needed.

This process transforms the protocol from a temporary plan into a way of living that adjusts naturally to your circumstances. It gives you ownership of your healing, teaching you how to respond to your body's signals long after the structured phases of the program are complete. With this foundation, health stops feeling fragile and begins to feel dependable — not because symptoms never return, but because you know exactly how to meet them when they do.

Next-Level Tools and Professional Support

Once foundational habits are in place and your body begins to stabilize, advanced tools can help refine progress and uncover deeper insights. These are not shortcuts or replacements for lifestyle changes but amplifiers that provide clarity when self-observation alone cannot fully explain lingering symptoms. Choosing the right tools requires discernment; not every test or device is necessary, and the goal is always targeted action rather than chasing data for its own sake.

Functional Lab Testing

Traditional medicine often relies on standard blood panels to detect disease but may miss subtler imbalances that contribute to fatigue, inflammation, or hormonal disruption. Functional lab testing offers a more detailed look at how systems are performing, even when conventional markers appear normal. Examples include comprehensive stool analyses that reveal gut microbiome health, hormone panels that track cortisol rhythms and thyroid conversion, or nutrient tests that identify deficiencies impacting energy and mood.

These tests can be particularly useful when symptoms persist despite adherence to a protocol. For instance, ongoing digestive discomfort may point to hidden food sensitivities or microbial imbalances that basic elimination diets fail to uncover. Similarly, unresolved fatigue might stem from thyroid or adrenal patterns not visible on standard screenings. Guided interpretation by a qualified practitioner ensures results are applied in context rather than becoming overwhelming or misleading.

Biofeedback and Wearable Technology

Beyond lab work, certain tools allow real-time feedback on how lifestyle choices affect recovery. Heart rate variability monitors, sleep trackers, and continuous glucose monitors provide objective data about stress response, sleep quality, and blood sugar fluctuations. Used wisely, they highlight patterns you might miss — such as how late meals affect overnight rest or how specific foods influence energy crashes.

These devices should enhance awareness rather than create obsession. The aim is to learn trends that inform decisions, not to chase perfect numbers. For many, short-term use is enough to identify key patterns, after which reliance can decrease as intuition improves.

Working with professionals can make these advanced tools far more effective. A skilled practitioner helps interpret results in the context of your overall health rather than focusing on isolated numbers. For example, a functional medicine provider might review hormone testing alongside sleep habits, nutrition, and stress levels, connecting patterns that a single test result could not explain on its own. This integrated view prevents unnecessary interventions and focuses on practical, evidence-based adjustments.

Deciding when to seek professional support often depends on two factors: the persistence of symptoms and the limits of self-guided approaches. If fatigue, digestive issues, or inflammation continue despite consistent lifestyle changes, advanced evaluation may reveal hidden drivers such as nutrient malabsorption, hormonal imbalances, or chronic infections. Professional guidance is also valuable when symptoms are complex, involving multiple systems at once, or when health goals extend beyond general well-being into performance optimization or long-term disease prevention.

Cost and accessibility should also be considered. Many advanced tests and interventions are not covered by insurance and can quickly become expensive. Prioritizing foundational habits first ensures you invest in these tools only when necessary rather than using them as substitutes for consistent daily practices. When chosen thoughtfully, a single well-timed test can clarify months of uncertainty, allowing you to target your efforts with precision rather than trial and error.

Avoiding over-testing is equally important. In the search for answers, it is tempting to run every available panel or try every new technology, but too much data can create confusion instead of clarity. A focused approach — guided by symptoms, progress tracking, and professional insight — ensures that information serves healing rather than overwhelming it.

Ultimately, advanced tools and professional support should enhance, not replace, your relationship with your own body. They provide valuable snapshots of internal processes but cannot capture everything that matters — the subtle improvements in energy, the ease of waking rested, the calm that comes from feeling steady in daily life. Combining personal awareness with selective testing creates a balanced path forward: informed by science, grounded in experience, and adaptable as your needs evolve.

This integration marks the final step in personalizing your healing journey. With foundational habits established and deeper insights available when needed, you gain both confidence and flexibility. You are no longer dependent on protocols alone but equipped with a framework to navigate any stage of life with clarity and resilience.

Last Words: Thank You

Thank you for reading this book and choosing to invest in your health in a world that often makes it complicated.

The changes you've learned here are not about perfection, trends, or chasing quick fixes. They are about remembering how capable your body is of healing when it is supported instead of fought against.

If you take only one thing with you, let it be this: **you are not broken.** Your body's signals — the fatigue, the inflammation, the brain fog — were never betrayals. They were requests for help. And by listening to them, you've already taken the first and most important step toward lasting change.

Healing is not linear. Some days will feel easier than others, and that is okay. The point is not to avoid every setback, but to know you can come back from them stronger and wiser. Over time, the daily choices you make will add up to something far greater than a "protocol" — they will become a way of living that sustains you for life.

Thank you for allowing me to share this path with you. May it help you feel clearer, stronger, and more alive than you thought possible.

www.ingramcontent.com/pod-product-compliance
Lightning Source LLC
Chambersburg PA
CBHW052211270326
41931CB00011B/2310